Maximum Hoof Power

ALSO BY CHERRY HILL

101 Horsemanship and Equitation Patterns
Stablekeeping
Trailering Your Horse
Longeing and Long Lining the English and Western Horse
101 Longeing and Long Lining Exercises, English and Western
Beginning English Exercises
Intermediate English Exercises
Advanced English Exercises
Beginning Western Exercises
Intermediate Western Exercises
Advanced Western Exercises
Horse Health Care
Horse Handling and Grooming
Your Pony, Your Horse
Horse for Sale
101 Arena Exercises
Horseowner's Guide to Lameness (with Dr. Ted S. Stashak)
Making Not Breaking
Becoming an Effective Rider
Horsekeeping on a Small Acreage
From the Center of the Ring
The Formative Years

Maximum Hoof Power
A Horse Owner's Guide to Shoeing and Soundness

Cherry Hill and Richard Klimesh, CJF

Trafalgar Square Publishing

NORTH POMFRET, VERMONT

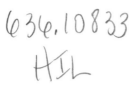

This paperback edition first published in 2000 by
Trafalgar Square Publishing, North Pomfret, Vermont 05053

First published in 1994 by Howell Book House, Macmillan Publishing Company,
New York, New York

Photographs by Cherry Hill on pages 129, 130 and 152 reprinted from *Becoming an Effective Rider* ©
1991 by Cherry Hill, published by Storey Communications, Inc., Pownal, Vermont. Illustrations by
N.J. Wiley on pages 83, 91, 100, 141, and 142 reprinted from *From the Center of the Ring* © 1988 by
Cherry Hill, published by Storey Communications, Inc., Pownal, Vermont.

Photographs by Cherry Hill and Richard Klimesh unless otherwise noted.

Illustrations by Peggy Judy unless otherwise noted.

Disclaimer of Liability: The authors and publisher shall have neither liability nor responsibility to
any person or entity with respect to any loss or damage caused or alleged to be caused directly or
indirectly by the information contained in this book. While the book is as accurate as the authors
can make it, there may be errors, omissions, and inaccuracies.

Library of Congress Cataloging-in-Publication Data
Hill, Cherry, 1947-
    Maximum hoof power : a horse owner's guide to shoeing and soundness / Cherry Hill and
Richard Klimesh.
    p. cm.
      Originally published: New York : Howell Book House, 1994.
      Includes bibliographical references (p.).
      ISBN 1-57076-168-X (pbk.)
      1. Hoofs—Care and hygiene. 2. Horseshoeing. I. Klimesh, Richard. II. Title.
    SF907 .H54 2000
    636.1'0833—dc21   00-026403
                                                                  CIP

Cover design by Carrie Fradkin

10 9 8 7 6 5 4 3 2 1

Printed in Canada

For my mom, Helen, who gave me life, taught me to laugh and encouraged me to be who I am.

RICHARD KLIMESH

For my mom, Sally, who is one of my best friends.

CHERRY HILL

We also dedicate this book to conscientious horse owners and farriers everywhere.

RICHARD AND CHERRY

Contents

Part Three Teamwork

Acknowledgments

Our thanks to the following people for their contributions of ideas and photos: Al Cook Al Dunning Breakthrough Publications Brenda Pieper Carla Wennberg Charlie Brown Chip Capobianco D. Kay Klein Dan Hubbell Dan Verniero Dave Remley Dick Pieper Dr. J. Frank Gravlee Dr. Olin Balch Dr. Ted S. Stashak Garden Way Publishing Hidden Hill Arabians Jas McMahon Jeff Rodriguez Jim Clanin John McConnell Kathleen Donnelly Les Vogt Lynn Brown Margot Dippert Midge Ames Mike Carlson Paige Tomberlin Patty Arnette RaeAnn Curtis Red Renchin Robert S. Hess Russ Jensen Sue Dixon Susan Wallen Sweet Briar College Terry Escher Tish Quirk Valerie Parry

Preface

Today's number one horse training and performance goal is longevity. Since it takes a great deal of time and emotional involvement to develop an equine athlete, it is heartbreaking when an exceptionally talented and well-trained horse cannot perform due to an avoidable lameness. Keys to a long, active performance career include conscientious hoof care and the employment of *preventive* shoeing by a qualified farrier whose priorities are balance, support and natural movement.

Through the years, I have often seen hooves that are desperately in need of proper hoof care: long-toed, low-heeled hooves that have collapsed over their shoes. These hooves appear on horses in all types of work, but, oddly, they are often seen on fat, gleaming horses that are sporting several thousand dollars' worth of tack and attire.

Ironically, some horses manage to perform fairly well when they are young, in spite of improper or irregular hoof care. But a horse forced to use unbalanced hooves or unsupported limbs usually fades away long before he reaches his prime. He may become so lame that he must be "retired" early. Or his chronic low-level discomfort may cause him to have an overall bad attitude toward his work.

Once you get a horse solidly trained, don't you want to enjoy him for a long time? I do. There is nothing more satisfying than sitting on a sound, well-trained and fit horse that enjoys his work and is confident and comfortable in his movement. His performance might be lyrical or explosive, collected or flat out, delicate or powerful. But what all top-notch performances have in common is that the horse and rider are in balance and harmony, the work is correct, the atmosphere is one of cooperation and the dialogue is interactive and dynamic. Time and dedication are essential for such an experience, but even then all the details must be right. I've learned that two of the most important ingredients in the performance formula are proper hoof management and shoeing.

To extend your horse's useful life, to optimize his performance and to prevent lameness, take an active role in the care and management of his hooves. I hope that you have the opportunity to work with a good farrier and an experienced equine veterinarian and that together you can achieve maximum hoof power.

CHERRY HILL

The human-horse relationship has been a source of awe and inspiration for thousands of years. Today's farrier is in the very special position of being able to enhance this relationship more than ever before. He can help a horse survive and flourish in a modern domestic environment that is often far different from the natural environment of the horse's ancestors. A farrier can also help horse owners develop an equine partner with four sound hooves that allow him to perform his work confidently and comfortably.

A very rewarding aspect of my career is seeing one of my clients enjoying time with his or her horse, especially if I have been instrumental in improving the hooves. I am sometimes disappointed, however, when all of my interest and experience brings only marginal improvement in the condition of a horse's feet. Optimum hoof health is a team effort: the horse provides the hooves, you train the horse and manage his exercise and environment, and the farrier protects the hooves and trains them to grow in a correct form.

Finding the right farrier may be all that is necessary to help a horse reach his hoof potential. However, our super-technology has yet to develop a magic rasp that can evaporate the effects of poor management.

Providing a friendly environment for your horse's feet is one of your primary responsibilities. The first step toward this goal is learning what kind of environment is healthy for hooves. In most cases, it will not require anything dramatic to reach the "ideal" situation that will improve your horse's feet. At times your management may only require a few simple changes or routines, which we will share with you in this book.

Myths and misinformation concerning hoof care and horseshoeing continue to appear in popular magazines. One of our goals in this book is to replace the myths with sound ideas that will help your horse enjoy healthy hooves throughout his life. May the forge be with you.

RICHARD KLIMESH

This book is based on our collective years of observations and experiences. In addition, we have taken into consideration all contemporary works on hoof care, shoeing, and movement, including research papers and articles that describe the concepts of the world's top veterinarians and farriers. We have also discussed our ideas with equine veterinarians specializing in lameness as well as knowledgeable farriers and prominent trainers across the country.

RICHARD and CHERRY

PART ONE

Shoeing Demystified

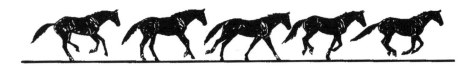

Old Mares' Tales

Old notions survive because few people question them. They are passed along from one generation to another whether they are based on fact or anecdote. Horseshoeing has an unhealthy share of old mares' tales that need to be whisked away. Some of them have had such a negative effect on horses' hooves, limbs and performance over the years that we feel the best way to open our book is by dispelling the myths.

If you want to score an easy 100% on a true/false test, here's your chance. Just answer false to each of the following statements and you're automatically an A + student. However, what's most important is to understand *why* these statements are false. We refute each myth and then refer you to the chapters that offer you more information.

- *Overflow the water trough because it is good for a horse to stand in mud.* Actually, mud and excess moisture are two of the biggest culprits that cause cracks, thrush, white line disease, poor hoof quality and lost shoes. See Chapters 11, 14 and 15.
- *The ideal hoof angle is 45 degrees.* Do you want to hear your farrier laugh? Just ask him when the last time his hoof gauge measured a 45-degree hoof. Although textbooks have long touted 45 as an ideal, the angles of normal, healthy hooves are much steeper. Forcing a horse to "be a 45 when he's really a 54" can cause devastating problems. See Chapters 3, 5 and 11.
- *A long toe lengthens and softens a horse's stride.* In the past, racehorses, hunters, Western Pleasure horses and even reining horses were shod with long toes to supposedly gain a performance advantage. Usually all that was gained were navicular problems and tendon strain. Recent research has disproved the myth of the long-toe advantage. See Chapters 5, 7 and 11.

- *A hoof with cracks is too dry.* Actually, in most cases, hoof cracks indicate just the opposite—the hoof has been too wet! See Chapters 11, 14 and 15.
- *Hoof dressing adds moisture and nutrients to the hoof wall, thereby improving hoof quality.* Most moisture is delivered to the hoof internally from the blood, so regular exercise will add more moisture to the hoof than hoof dressing. And the thick outer hoof is essentially "dead" tissue anyway, so it cannot utilize any supposed "nutrients" from hoof dressing. See Chapter 14.
- *Black hooves are better than white hooves.* According to research, there is no difference in hardness, toughness or brittleness. See Chapter 3.
- *The frog must contact the ground in order for the blood to circulate in the hoof properly.* The frogs are not "extra hearts" or "blood pumps" as they have often been called over the years. In fact, in a healthy hoof the frog does not have to be in contact with the ground for the hoof to function properly. See Chapter 3.
- *Horses that aren't ridden frequently don't need to be shod as often as those that are ridden regularly.* Whether a horse is ridden or not, his hooves are growing at a certain rate, and that is what dictates the need for reshoeing. See Chapters 4 and 5.
- *All horses should be allowed to go barefoot for part of the year.* A healthy hoof that is properly shod does not *need* to go barefoot. Routinely "pulling the shoes for the winter" can be very harmful to hooves that require shoes for protection and support. It can take several shoeing periods to restore a hoof that was damaged in a few days. Some hooves can maintain soundness without shoes; but they, too, will likely require regular trimming. See Chapter 4.
- *Mud will suck a horseshoe right off a hoof.* If you have ever tried to remove a properly applied shoe without first opening the clinches, you know the tremendous amount of force that mud would have to exert to suck off a shoe. To get a different perspective on the mud myth, see Chapters 5, 8 and 15.
- *The best shoeing job is the one that stays on the longest.* In fact, the best shoeing job may be the one that comes off easily! Shoes that are fit very close and nailed very securely to the foot often compromise the long-term health of the hoof. See Chapters 5 and 15.
- *Shoeing is a necessary evil.* This one really hurts a conscientious farrier every time it's said. Good shoeing can be one of the greatest gifts you give to your horse. It will not only make him more comfortable but also increase his useful life as well. See Chapters 4 and 5.

Your Questions Answered

To further demystify horseshoeing, here are the questions commonly asked by horse owners at seminars and during shoeing appointments. The working farrier may not be in a position to give a thorough answer because he is often crouched under a 1,200-pound equine and has a mouthful of nails! Following the brief answers are additional references.

- *Does it hurt a horse to have his feet trimmed or shod?* When performed in a proper manner, trimming and shoeing cause a horse no discomfort. Lame, sick, very old or arthritic horses or mares late in gestation may be somewhat uncomfortable standing on three legs for long periods. Hoof trimming itself is similar to nail clipping, painless because only insensitive tissue is removed. Properly driven nails contact insensitive tissue only. However, when a nail is driven too close to sensitive tissue, or if the sole is trimmed too thin, the horse will experience pain. See Chapters 5 and 11.
- *Wild horses don't need shoes. Why do we have to shoe our domestic horses?* Domestic horses are often confined to environments that are not hoof-friendly. In addition, domestic horses are usually required to carry the weight of a rider and tack. While natural selection of wild horses favors individuals with healthy, tough feet, the artificial selection imposed by humans often selects for small hooves or ignores hoof shape and quality altogether to concentrate on cosmetic traits. The vast, dry, natural environment afforded wild horses produces much stronger, healthier hooves than most domestic management situations. See Chapters 4 and 14.
- *Why does my horse misbehave when my farrier is shoeing him?* A horse must learn a specific progression of proper shoeing manners,

just as he learns certain lessons to be ridden. Many horses have not had formal training in tying, restraint, leg handling and balancing on three legs for extended periods of time. Because they have not learned what is expected of them, they are insecure and "misbehave." See Chapters 4 and 14.

- *Why does my farrier insist on shoeing my horse every six weeks when I know his shoes will last for twelve?* It is the growth of the hoof that determines the time for rebalancing, not the number of weeks or the wear on the shoe. Your farrier's education and experience allow him to determine the optimum time to shoe your horse in order to prevent problems from occurring. See Chapters 4, 5 and 11.

- *Is hot shoeing better than cold shoeing?* Hot shoeing means that the shoe is either made from scratch in a forge or a factory-made shoe is heated in a forge to be shaped and/or fit to the hoof. Cold shoeing simply means the farrier shapes and applies the shoe without heating it up. If good horseshoeing principles are followed, both methods yield satisfactory results. See Chapters 5 and 6.

- *Wouldn't it be best for my horse to have new shoes every time he is shod?* Not necessarily. Sometimes it is better for your farrier to reset the same shoes. See Chapter 5.

- *Why are only six nails used when there are eight nail holes in a horseshoe?* Nails should generally be placed forward of the widest part of the hoof because the hoof grows wider as it grows longer and it also expands and contracts with each step. In most factory-made shoes, the two nail holes nearest the heel are behind the widest part of the hoof, so nails used in these holes would restrict natural growth and movement of the hoof. See Chapter 5.

- *My horse has been diagnosed "navicular." Is there any hope of ever using him again?* Many horses suffering from navicular syndrome respond positively to proper shoeing and return to their previous level of performance. See Chapter 11.

- *Should I use hoof dressing, and if so, what kind and how often?* Hoof dressing is generally not necessary for healthy hooves, and too much hoof dressing can soften and weaken hooves. In many cases, however, a hoof *sealer* is beneficial. See Chapter 14.

- *I recently saw horseshoes for sale in one of my tack catalogs: 4 shoes for $6. Why does my farrier charge $80 to shoe my horse and the same amount even when he reuses the same shoes?* Farriers are self-employed professionals whose rates reflect the time they have invested in their education as well as their level of skill and experience. From the $80, your farrier must maintain and replace his tools and truck (his shop on wheels); buy gas, oil and insurance (truck, health, disability and liability); pay self-employment tax; finance his continuing education through seminars and journals; fund his retirement; save a little for a vacation (if he ever takes one); pay normal family living expenses, and buy a cup of coffee to get him to the next farm. *Now* doesn't $80 sound like a bargain? See Chapters 5 and 16.

- *My horse is always losing shoes. Is this the farrier's fault?* Lost shoes can be related to something that a farrier is doing wrong, but ironically they can also occur because the farrier is doing everything very, very right! Lost shoes can be the result of many factors, from the horse's conformation to your riding. See Chapters 8, 9 and 15.
- *What is the difference between a horseshoer, a farrier and a blacksmith?* A horseshoer puts shoes on horses. A farrier is a horseshoer who prefers to be called a farrier. A blacksmith uses a forge and anvil to fashion items from steel. A hundred years ago, a blacksmith not only made horseshoes but also applied them to horses, so to this day some people (erroneously) refer to horseshoers and farriers as blacksmiths. See Chapters 5 and 16.

C H A P T E R   3

Foot Works

Why do some horses move crisply and boldly while others dawdle
or move meekly and cautiously? Why do some horses develop
and maintain a generous, healthy hoof while other horses' hooves
become smaller and contracted? What makes some hooves tough and
durable and others brittle and pithy? The answers begin with a basic
knowledge of how the foot works. For more detailed information on
equine anatomy, refer to the Recommended Reading list in the Appendix.

The term *hoof* refers to the horny external material making up the
hoof wall, sole and frog. The term *foot* includes the hoof and its
internal structures. The internal structures include the bones, the
sensitive structures, the insensitive structures and the elastic structures.

Although the anatomical directional terms *dorsal* and *palmar*
(*plantar* for the hind) are the most correct when talking about the
front and back of a horse's hoof and lower limb, the terms *anterior-
posterior* and *cranial-caudal* have also been used.

The most distal bone, which is hoof-shaped, has been referred to
by many names: the coffin bone, pedal bone, distal phalanx, third
phalanx, PIII and "P-3." Located between the wings of the coffin bone
is the navicular bone, sometimes referred to as the distal sesamoid
bone. The flexor tendons connect the flexor muscles of the upper limb
to the bones of the lower limb. The deep digital flexor tendon inserts
on the palmar (and plantar) surface of the coffin bone. The superficial
flexor tendon inserts on the distal end of the long pastern bone and
the proximal end of the short pastern bone.

The short pastern bone articulates with the coffin bone and the

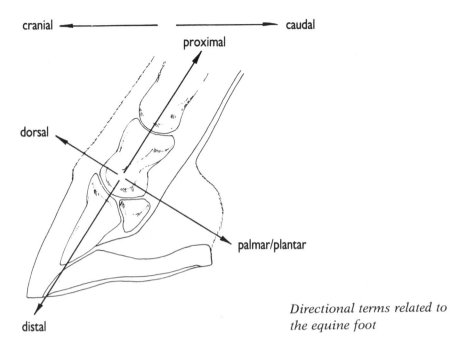

cranial ←—————— ——————→ caudal

proximal

dorsal

palmar/plantar

distal

Directional terms related to the equine foot

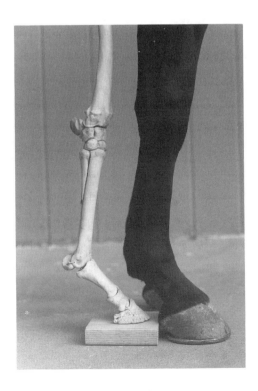

Lower leg bones

navicular bone at the coffin joint. The pastern joint is formed at the junction of the short pastern bone and long pastern bone. The fetlock is formed by the junction of the long pastern bone, the distal end of the cannon bone and the two (proximal) sesamoid bones.

It is important to distinguish between the terms *cannon* and *cannon bone*. *Cannon bone* is an anatomical term that refers only to the long bone between the knee and the fetlock. *Cannon* is a conformational term that refers to the area between the knee and fetlock, which includes the cannon bone, flexor and extensor tendons, suspensory ligament, soft tissues and skin. This distinction is significant in understanding shoeing guidelines that are outlined in Chapter 5.

The hoof is lined with corium (popularly called the quick), a sensitive, blood-rich tissue that nourishes the horn-producing structures of the foot, provides moisture to the hoof wall and keeps the foot warm via blood flow. The corium is sub-named according to the outer structure it nourishes such as coronary corium, perioplic corium, laminar corium, sole corium and frog corium. The majority of hoof growth (approximately 70%) occurs at the coronary band; however, a significant contribution (approximately 30%) is made by the dermal (sensitive) laminae.

Depending on the horse, diet, exercise and season, hoof growth rates can vary from 0 to 1/2 inch per month. The average is 1/4 inch per month. It takes six to eight months (five shoeing periods) on the average for new hoof, created at the coronet, to reach the normal nailing area. Hoof growth slows during the winter months and increases in the spring and summer. Regular exercise increases the blood flow in the foot and usually results in faster hoof growth.

The corium also serves to attach the hoof to the rest of the foot. The laminar corium attaches to the wall of the coffin bone and provides nourishment for the dermal (sensitive) laminae. The dermal (sensitive) laminae interlock with the epidermal (insensitive) laminae, which line the interior of the hoof capsule. Rather than sitting on the sole, the coffin bone is suspended by the laminae attached to the hoof wall. The Velcro-like attachment of the laminae must be very strong, as it is responsible for bearing the entire weight of the horse.

The insensitive structures are identifiable externally. The bars are a portion of the hoof wall that angle forward from the heels and toward each side of the frog. The sole is the hornlike material covering the bottom of the hoof. A well-conformed sole should be cupped so it doesn't readily contact a flat ground surface.

The frog is the V-shaped cushion located between the heels on the ground surface of the hoof. The collateral clefts separate the frog from the bars. The frog helps provide traction to the hoof and protects the

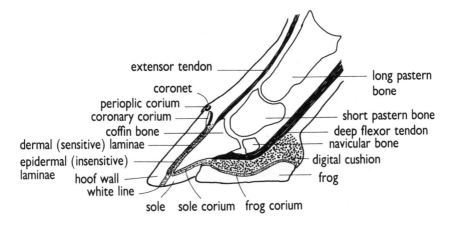

Some of the internal parts of the equine foot.
Richard Klimesh drawing

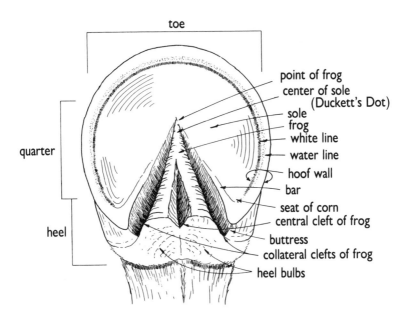

The external parts of an equine hoof. Richard Klimesh drawing

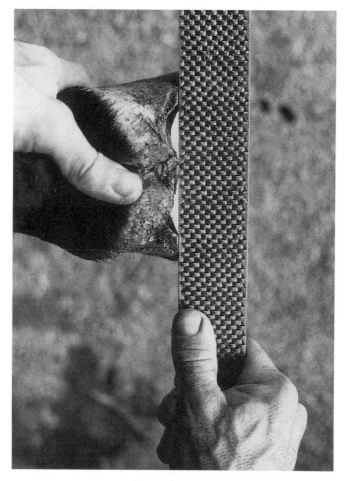

Frog clearance

sensitive inner structures of the hoof while allowing the hoof capsule to expand and contract. It also acts as a shock absorber, but it is not necessary or desirable for the frog to contact or bear weight on flat ground. The majority of the weight of the horse should be borne by the wall.

The hoof wall is comprised of three layers, listed from external to internal: (1) the periople/tectorum; (2) tubules; (3) epidermal (insensitive) laminae. The periople is a narrow strip above the coronary band that functions somewhat like the human cuticle. The periople produces a waxy protective coating that migrates down the hoof and, in essence, becomes the tectorum, a very thin keratin layer that gives a healthy hoof its natural glossy appearance.

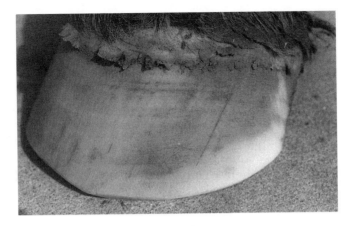

Periople

The tubules are the fibers that make up the bulk of the hoof wall. In a well-conformed hoof, the tubules run parallel to each other and perpendicular to the coronary band, which is the strongest configuration. The angle of the tubules is more easily seen in a black-and-white-striped hoof. Studies involving domestic and wild horses have indicated that there is no apparent structural difference between pigmented and nonpigmented hooves. Hoof horn tubules are hollow and capable of containing moisture.

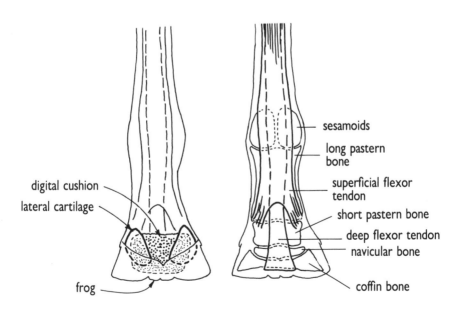

Equine foot structures from the rear. Richard Klimesh drawing

As mentioned, the epidermal (insensitive) laminae connect the hoof to the dermal (sensitive) laminae of the coffin bone. Normally, the weight of the horse does not pass from the coffin bone to the sole but is transmitted via the laminae to the wall.

The elastic structures are involved in absorbing concussion. The lateral cartilages are located on each side of the rear of the coffin bone. The top edge of the lateral cartilages extend above the coronary band and can be felt as pliable, resilient structures in young horses and hard structures in many old, sound horses or those with sidebone. The lateral cartilages help to fasten the hoof wall to the coffin bone. The digital cushion is a thick, fibrous, fatty pad located between the coffin bone and the frog/sole. It extends rearward to support the bulbs of the heel.

The lateral cartilages, digital cushion and frog work together to absorb concussion. As weight descends on the foot, the digital cushion is compressed between the bones and the frog/sole, and it spreads out and puts pressure on the lateral cartilages and the walls (see figure on page 13). This causes the concave sole to momentarily flatten somewhat and the heels to spread (Chapter 5). Also, the deformation of the digital cushion within the relatively unyielding hoof capsule squeezes blood out of the foot and sends it up into the limb on its way back to the heart.

To Shoe or Not to Shoe

Whether or not your horse needs shoes depends on his hoof and limb conformation, his intended use and your management.

Shoeing and trimming fall into three categories; preventive, corrective, and therapeutic. *Preventive* trimming and shoeing is characterized by balance, support and protection. The goals of preventive shoeing are long-term soundness and performance longevity. *Corrective* trimming and shoeing consists of altering the hoof to affect stance or stride. Properly employed corrective farriery generally does not force a limb into an abnormal position, it allows the hoof and limb to attain a desirable configuration and achieve sound movement. *Therapeutic* shoeing is often a part of lameness treatment designed to protect and/or support a damaged hoof or limb or to prevent or encourage a particular movement until healing can take place. Corrective and therapeutic farriery may be helpful in the treatment of some lameness but may have no beneficial effect in others. Certain lamenesses are not affected by shoeing. Preventive shoeing, however, should be a part of every horse's routine hoof care program, and all domestic horses need regular trimming.

THE BAREFOOT HORSE

You may have heard the advice, "Pull his shoes and turn him out for the winter." Although this suggestion has merit in certain situations, for some horses such a plan would lead to chronic hoof problems. The practice gained popularity during the era of horse-powered agriculture in areas with long, hard winters when most of the driving teams were not kept in full work. Turning a shod horse out in a snow-covered corn field, plowed field, or winter pasture would have been an open invitation for lost shoes. Also, a horse shod with plain shoes usually has poorer traction in many footings than if he is barefoot. What's more, shod horses turned out and fed in a group are more likely to injure one another if they kick. So, to the turn-of-the-century Midwest draft horse manager, pulling the shoes for the winter made sense.

Today's horse management is characterized by year-round use, more confinement and individualized feeding. Yet for some reason many horse owners still feel they should adhere to the age-old practice to ensure hoof health. The common belief is that pulling the shoes allows the hooves to "spread out and breathe." In fact, what often happens is that the hooves "flatten out and break."

To determine whether barefoot is a viable option for your horse,

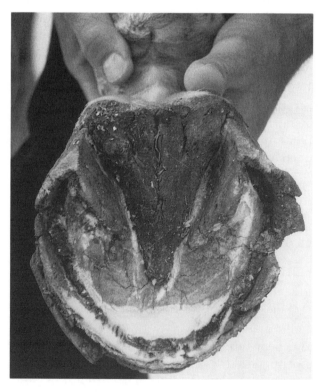

Broken and separated hoof wall

first weigh the advantages and disadvantages. Then evaluate your horse's hoof conformation to see if it resembles the "ideal" hoof that can go barefoot or the "problem" hoof that should not. Finally, take into consideration the additional management factors that may affect whether a horse can safely go barefoot.

Short-Term and Long-Term Costs

The primary advantage to letting a horse go barefoot is that it costs less in the short term. A hoof trim costs approximately one third or less of the price of a standard shoeing. However, to determine the overall savings netted from having a horse trimmed rather than shod during the winter months, you should take into account the *extra* farrier costs incurred the following spring, summer and fall that are the result of damage that occurred during the barefoot winter months.

It is not uncommon for a barefoot horse to be presented for his first spring shoeing with long toes, broken quarters, low heels, cracks and bruised soles. It may cost more in the long run for prosthetic hoof repair, clips, wedge pads and therapeutic shoeing for cracks and bruises than it would have if the horse had been kept shod all winter.

The Bare Advantages

A properly trimmed unshod hoof is easier to maintain as it more easily self-cleans than a shod hoof. Horseshoes tend to hold manure, mud, rocks and snow in the hoof cavity, which can put undesirable pressure on the sole and provide a favorable environment for the growth of anaerobic thrush bacteria. Horseshoes also trap moisture between the shoe and the ends of the hoof wall tubules and in some cases never allow the hoof to completely dry. In addition, mud, sand and water can be forced up into the weak areas of the hoof wall by the hydraulic pressure created when the shod hoof bears weight in deep, wet footing. In contrast, the rounded edge of a sound (healthy), bare hoof wall can more readily release excess moisture and can better maintain an optimum moisture equilibrium. Therefore, the barefoot hoof, *if it is of the desirable type,* is theoretically a healthier hoof.

If thin, well-designed horseshoe nails are used properly and old nail holes in the hoof are filled, nails pose no real threat to the health of the hoof. However, when large nails are driven indiscriminately and old nail holes are left open to invasion by moisture, soil, and manure, the strength of the hoof wall suffers. So in the instance of *poor* shoeing, the barefoot horse may be better off. Bad shoeing is often worse than none at all.

The barefoot horse has better traction than the conventionally shod horse in some situations, such as on rocks, concrete or hard ice. However, such footing can cause excess wear of the bare hoof. Conventional shoeing decreases hoof wear and specialized shoeing is available to increase traction. However, shod horses, and especially those shod with borium, ice nails or calks (see Traction in this chapter) are potentially more dangerous to other horses and humans in the event of a kick or being stepped on. Barefoot horses are safer to others as well as to themselves. Also, a shod horse has the potential of stepping the shoe off or getting its shoe caught on a fence or halter, often resulting in injury.

An instance where the horse may benefit from going barefoot is seen with the horse that has been closely shod (nails far back on the hoof, clips) and/or short shod (using a shoe too small for the support of the hoof) for several shoeings. Going barefoot may allow this hoof to relax and spread. However, if the hoof structure is not strong enough to hold up without shoes, the horse may derive more benefit from being shod properly than from going barefoot.

The Shoeing Edge

The barefoot hoof should be properly trimmed approximately every six weeks. However, it can be very difficult to maintain the balance of a bare hoof. The bare hoof is not protected from hoof wall wear and often wears unevenly, throwing the hoof out of balance. The wall can wear so excessively that the horse is walking on his soles. This often results in sole bruises and sole abscesses.

It is difficult to meet a horse's specialized corrective, therapeutic or performance needs when he is barefoot. In the case of cracks, for example, a shoe can stabilize the hoof as it heals and grows an entire new balanced hoof comprised of solid horn. Other problems such as laminitis, navicular disease syndrome, underrun heels and fractured coffin bones are often hopeless to treat without the use of appropriate shoes.

The equine hoof evolved to carry the horse's own weight in a semiarid environment. The wild horse's free movement over dry terrain encouraged the hooves to become very tough and resistant to abrasion. Natural selection eliminated horses with unsound feet, but once human selection began to take over, horses with poor feet were protected and kept in the gene pool. Also, domestic horses are usually

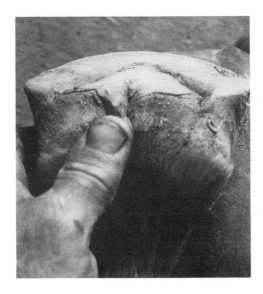

A short wall causes the sole to bear weight.

restricted to a small, moist environment that softens the hooves, allowing them to grow very long, deform and break off in chunks.

As man's dependence on the horse for transport and war decreased, it seems that emphasis on hoof quality also decreased. The domestic horse today often inherits poor feet, is fed too generously and is then required to perform carrying its overweight body plus an extra two hundred pounds of tack and rider. Appropriate shoes, knowledgeably applied, can help provide the support and comfort that will allow an overtaxed horse to be functional.

Evaluating Hoof Conformation

Barefoot candidates usually have an upright hoof and pastern axis, 54 degrees or greater. The heel angle is parallel to the toe angle, with minimal tendency to underrun heels. The hoof is free of dishes and flares; the wall is straight from the coronary band to the ground. The hoof horn is a high-quality material: thick, dense, hard and solid, yet resilient because of a proper balance between internal and external moisture. The hoof wall is thick through the quarters and into the heel. The bottom of the hoof is well cupped, with a durable yet resilient concave sole.

Unfortunately, most horses have hooves that are unsuitable for going barefoot in a domestic environment. Such hooves have the tendency to form long toes, low heels and underrun heels, where the heel angle is lower than the toe angle by 5 degrees or more. There are

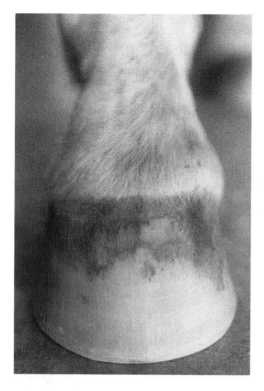

Barefoot candidate

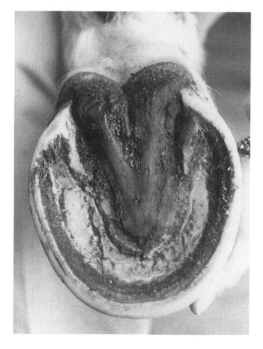

The hoof of a Trakehner stallion ridden barefoot in dressage

often dishes or flares, which can result in wall breakage. The hoof horn is weak: either soft, greasy or wet; brittle and chipping; hollow, pulpy or pithy. The hoof wall is thin and weak at the quarters and heels. The sole is flat or dropped (see photograph on page 19).

The hooves of wild horses are characteristically steeper than those of domestic horses (50 to 60 degrees in front and 53 to 63 behind). They exhibit a naturally rounded edge (perimeter), with the front hooves being rounder in shape, the hinds more pointed. The hooves are even, well-proportioned, balanced and symmetric. Wild horses are not a breed, but a mix of domestic horses living in a natural environment. Their freedom of movement over a dry, rugged terrain has much to do with their solid hoof qualities. It has been found that neither sex nor color of hoof has any obvious effect on hoof measurements or shape.

The young horse should go barefoot until factors indicate that he needs to be shod. Nailing shoes on foals for therapeutic reasons is difficult because of the small, thin-walled hooves. However, with the advent of glue-on shoes, foals as young as four weeks of age can safely be shod. Usually by twelve months of age, most horses have enough hoof to nail on a shoe if required for therapeutic reasons. However, if a young horse is going along all right without shoes, he can continue barefoot until activities require added support or protection.

The footing in which a horse works may allow him to permanently go barefoot. It is not uncommon to see barefoot dressage horses if they have good-quality hooves and are worked in a light, nonabrasive footing. However, most competitors, because they can never be sure what the footing will be at shows, keep their horses shod. If a work area or turnout area contains gravel, rocks or uneven ground, shoes will likely be required for protection and, in some cases, added traction. It is very uncommon to see a performance horse that is shod on the hinds and not on the fronts, as the front legs bear more weight and are the site of most limb and foot problems. Shoeing the fronts and leaving the hinds bare is not uncommon, especially for arena horses. However, if the hinds are allowed to wear too short or are too small to provide necessary support, the horse may become reluctant to bear weight with the hind legs and may not balance his weight rearward or drive energetically.

A horse that is too heavy for its hoof size may require shoes to help keep the hooves, especially of the front feet, from collapsing. Mares in foal, overweight horses and horses that have genetically small feet in relation to body size may be uncomfortable going barefoot. It is generally recommended for safety reasons that breeding stock involved

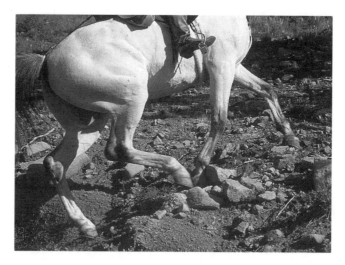

The hooves of this Arabian endurance horse require shoes for protection and traction.

in natural breeding be barefoot. It is especially important that the hinds of the mare and the fronts of the stallion either be barefoot or padded during breeding.

Although wild horses have survived in their own natural environment without farrier care, to make domestic horses comfortable and functional, most need regular and competent trimming and shoeing.

PURPOSES OF SHOEING

Protection In a domestic environment, the growth rate of a horse's hooves in relation to hoof wear is rarely equitable. The hooves either wear away faster than they grow and the horse is sore. Or the hooves grow faster than they wear, become very long, then crack or break out and the horse is lame. Shoes can protect the hooves from wear and breakage and allow the horse to function comfortably and remain sound. See Chapters 5, 6 and 10.

Maintain Balance A domestic environment drastically changes the horse's natural patterns and rhythms of movement. Consequently, the hooves often wear in an unbalanced fashion. This puts uneven stress on the support structures of the limb and can lead to lameness. Shoes can help to maintain the hoof balance and minimize unsoundness. See Chapters 5, 6 and 10.

TRACTION GUIDELINES

- Determine the activity level of the horse.
- Know the performance requirements.
- Consider the footing.
- Select the appropriate type of traction device.
- Apply traction devices very moderately at first.
- Use traction devices on both feet and on both sides of the shoe to prevent uneven torque.
- Gradually build up the traction to the optimum level.
- Closely monitor the horse for signs of stress.
- Realize that a small degree of slide upon landing is desirable, as it will dissipate some shock that would otherwise be transmitted to the horse's limb.

Provide Support Domestic breeding and unnatural environment have resulted in a greater number of horses that have feet either too small or too weak to hold up under the demands placed upon them. When the foundation of the horse breaks down, lameness is inevitable. Properly applied shoes can optimize the support of the limb and help hold the hoof together. See Chapters 5, 6 and 10.

Provide Traction To perform safely, confidently and without unnecessary exertion, a horse needs appropriate traction for his activity. Traction is covered in detail below.

Traction Principles

The barefoot horse has quite good traction in a variety of low-demand situations, especially if the hooves are naturally balanced, with dense hoof horn and a well-cupped sole. Such a hoof is able to grip most surfaces without hoof damage, and the naturally concave sole sheds mud and slush well. In contrast, a bare hoof with a long toe and low heel, brittle or pithy horn and a flat sole does not have adequate traction. If you think of the ideal hoof as contacting the ground somewhat like a suction cup, the poor hoof would be more like a stale pancake.

A horse's traction requirements will depend on his use (Chapter 10) and the footing (Chapter 8). In some instances, a horse needs greater traction than would be provided by a plain keg shoe (Chapter 6). The types of shoes and nails used and the addition of borium or calks can increase traction. Optimum traction can increase horse and rider safety, increase a horse's feeling of security so he will stride normally, help a horse to maintain his balance in unstable footing such as mud, ice, snow or rock and minimize fatigue.

Before you consider using traction devices, be sure your horse is fit and in working condition. A thorough conditioning program should do more than increase a horse's cardiopulmonary (heart-lung) efficiency. It should toughen the ligaments and condition (via progressive, regulated stretching and strengthening exercises) the muscles and tendons.

Moderation Traction should be added moderately. Using excess traction or suddenly applying devices unfamiliar to a horse may cause him to exert dangerous stresses on his muscles, tendons, bones, ligaments and joints. The structures in the limbs only have the capacity to take a certain amount of torque before something is damaged, no matter how fit a horse is. Torque is the twisting force that occurs when the horse's leg is subjected to opposing forces. A horse with too much traction would be like you taking country swing lessons in golf shoes on carpet.

A hoof (or foot) normally goes through a certain amount of slide and often some degree of rotation as it lands and gets ready to take off again. If a horse is deprived of this normal motion (suddenly or excessively), the forces are taken up by the joints and tendons. Injuries from excessive or inappropriate traction can show up immediately or after long-term use.

A horse also needs to *mentally* become accustomed to his new grab on the ground. He needs to be relaxed enough to devise new ways to balance his body to compensate for the change in his traction. Sometimes a jumper may have the confidence to negotiate a tight turn "off balance" if he knows he won't slip and can readily regain his balance with good ground contact. This results in a faster turn but also has the potential for greater trauma to his legs.

On the other hand, requiring a horse to work on precarious footing without adequate traction can result in muscle strain (such as in the gluteals and hamstrings) caused by constant slipping. Therefore, the goal is to supply enough traction to get the job done safely but no extra. Finding the optimum amount of traction that is required for your particular activity and specific footing is something a qualified farrier is trained to do.

Use Traction Bilaterally Borium spots or smears, ice nails and calks should always be applied on both sides of a shoe (and on both shoes of a pair of legs) to prevent uneven torque on landing or takeoff. (There are times when the judicious application of only one traction

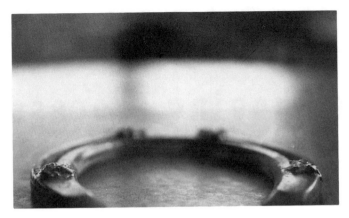

Borium spots for traction

device on a shoe or two different devices on the same shoe might be warranted for correcting a travel defect.)

Customarily ice nails are applied at the third nail-hole position, at the midpoint of each side of the shoe. This results in the safest grab with minimal torque. If four calks are used on a shoe, two are placed just ahead of the toe nails and two in the heel area. If only two are used, they are located either at the heels or at the midpoint of the shoe. Borium is usually added just ahead of both toe nails and just behind each heel nail.

Monitor for Signs of Stress When a horse realizes that his hooves are going to stick rather than land, slide and twist, he will be able to adjust his balance and movement accordingly. As traction is increased, it is important to stay within an individual horse's limits of tolerance. The goal is *optimum* traction, not *maximum* traction. Finding out what is ideal requires some fine tuning and detective work.

Know the warning signs of excessive traction: lameness, swelling, heat, a reluctance to work, a shortened stride, a bad attitude. All of these can indicate that a horse is trying to protect himself. Contrary to what is commonly thought, tendons can only stretch about 3% of their length. Exceeding this elastic range can bring detrimental changes to the mechanical characteristics of the tendon fibers. Ligaments have almost no ability to stretch, so when they are wrenched, it usually results in a tear.

If you are thinking about adding traction to your horse's shoes, discuss it thoroughly with your farrier. Be sure you know the requirements of your sport, choose appropriate traction devices, use them conservatively and monitor your horse's reaction to them carefully.

C H A P T E R 5

The Shoeing Process

Each farrier has a customary routine for removing shoes, evaluating hooves and shoeing. By describing one process, we do not suggest that alternate ways of doing things are not correct. Many farriers are fine craftsmen who devise custom ways of performing their work. The following guidelines are offered to help you get an overall feel for the process.

Before removing the old shoes, the farrier often discusses problems or concerns the owner or trainer has related to the horse's movement. If the horse is a regular client, the farrier probably has notes about previous shoeings. With routine shoeing, movement evaluation is not usually necessary, but in new or problem cases (Chapter 9) it helps if the farrier sees the horse ridden by his usual rider in customary footing. Alternatively, the owner may be asked to lead the horse at a walk and trot in a straight line so the farrier can evaluate the movement from the front, rear and side. When dealing with a gait abnormality, a video camera may be used as part of the evaluation procedure (Chapters 7 and 9).

The farrier is primarily interested in how the hoof lands, settles and breaks over. The hoof should land flat or very slightly heel first but generally not toe first. If the hoof is not landing properly at time of reset, it could indicate that the hoof was not correctly shod in the first place, the hoof has grown out of balance since the last shoeing, the horse is adjusting to pain or the horse's conformation is such that the hoof simply does not land flat.

An experienced farrier can often tell by the wear of the shoe and the shape of the hoof how to proceed with the trimming and shoeing. Most horses require shoeing every five to eight weeks to prevent the increasing width of the hoof from exceeding the fixed width of the shoe. Also, the hoof wall at the toe grows faster than that at the heel, which requires the hoof to be rebalanced.

If the horse is to be left barefoot, the farrier will trim the hoof to minimize breakage and ensure balance. If the horse is to be reshod, the farrier will examine each hoof and shoe for clues to the horse's individual wear patterns. With the shoe off, the hoof angle can be determined using a hoof gauge, and the length of the untrimmed hoof can be measured with dividers or a ruler. The farrier will assess balance, shape and symmetry. He will look for the tendency of the hoof to form flares or dishes. He will evaluate the symmetry of the hoof in relationship to the bulbs of the heels and the lower limb.

Next the farrier will pare the sole, nip or rasp the hoof wall, trim any excess frog and dress (rasp) the outside of the hoof wall if it has

---

HOW TO REMOVE A SHOE

Use the following procedure to remove a shoe that has become bent or dangerously loose, or has rotated on your horse's hoof.

Necessary tools, from left: clinch cutter, hammer, pull-offs, and crease nail puller.

Using the chisel end of the clinch cutter, open the clinches by tapping the spine of the clinch cutter with the hammer. A clinch is the end of the nail folded over; this needs to be opened so that the nails can slide straight through the hoof wall when pulled without taking large hunks of hoof with them.

If the shoe has a crease on the bottom, you may be able to use the crease nail puller to extract each nail individually, allowing the shoe to come off. Nails with protruding heads can be pulled out using the pull-offs.

If you can't pull the nails out individually, then you will have to remove the shoe with the pull-offs. After the clinches have been opened, grab a shoe heel and pry *toward* the tip of the frog. Do the same with the other shoe heel.

When both heels are loose, grab one side of the shoe at the toe and pry toward the tip of the frog. Repeat around the shoe until it is removed. *Never* pry toward the outside of the hoof or you risk ripping big chunks out of the hoof wall. As the nail heads protrude from the loosening of the shoe, you can pull them out individually with the pull-offs.

Pull any nails that may remain in the hoof.

To protect the hoof until the shoe is replaced, wrap the hoof edges with tape, or if your horse has a tender sole, tape a cloth over the bottom of the hoof or use a protective boot. Keep the horse confined in soft bedding.

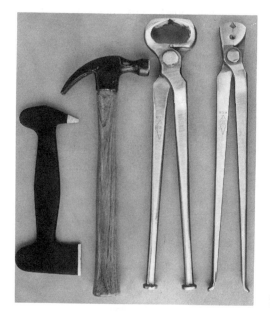

Tools for removing a shoe

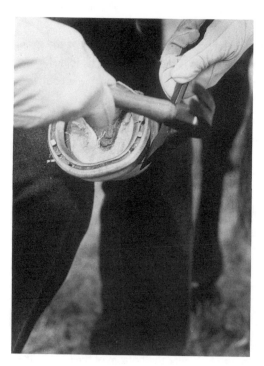

Opening a clinch

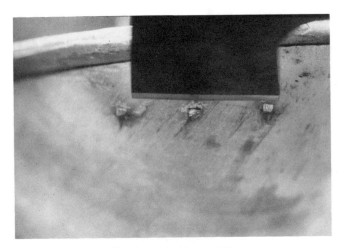

Clinch cutter in position

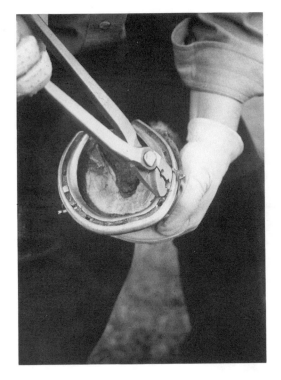

Using a crease nail puller

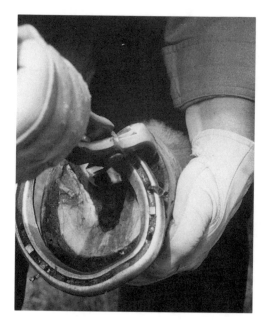

Using the pull-offs

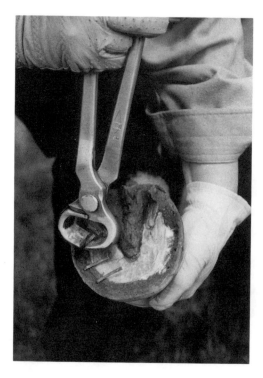

Removing remaining nails

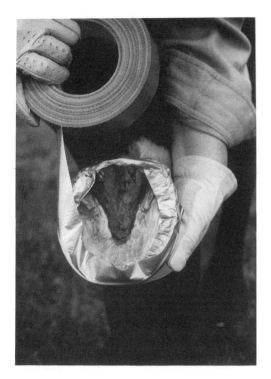

Taping a hoof

flares or dishes (see photograph on page 35). He will remeasure the hoof angle and length and evaluate the shape, balance and straightness of the hoof wall. When he is satisfied the hoof is ready, he will select the proper size and type of shoe for the horse. Many farriers prepare both hooves of a pair before nailing on a shoe. This allows him to make adjustments between the hooves to match angle and length.

A good farrier shapes a shoe to fit a properly prepared hoof, not the other way around. Generally it is a good sign if once the farrier has begun shaping the shoe he does not reshape the hoof with a rasp. Once he is satisfied with the fit of the shoe and the way it seats on the hoof wall, he will round any edges of the shoe that will be exposed. Then he will begin nailing.

Often he will drive two nails, wring off or bend over the sharp tips and set the hoof down to see how the shoe is positioned on the hoof. He will then drive the remaining nails and wring off or bend over the tips. After the nails have been driven, the clinches are set, blocked or tightened and filed or cut to a short consistent length. The clinches are then folded flat against the hoof wall and filed smooth.

The farrier may apply a hoof sealer to maintain the moisture bal-

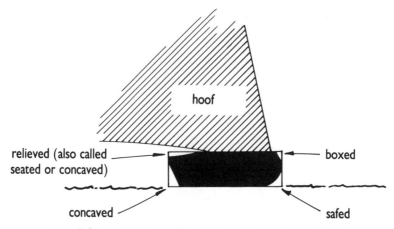

Modifications made to shoe edges. Richard Klimesh
drawing

ance of the hoof, especially if he has had to rasp the outer surface of
the hoof wall to remove flares or dishes. He may also use wax or
another substance to fill old nail holes as well as the new ones. This
will prevent mud, urine and water from invading the hoof and causing cracks.

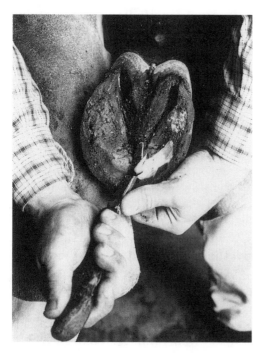

Trimming the sole

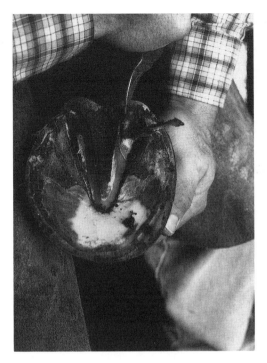

Trimming the frog

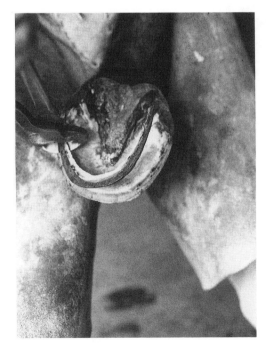

Nipping the hoof wall

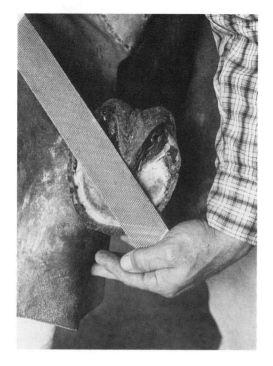

Rasping the bottom of the hoof

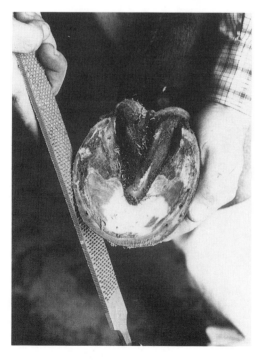

Shaping the hoof

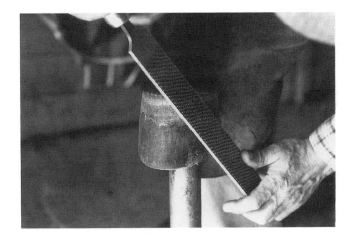

Dressing a flare

Checking for dish

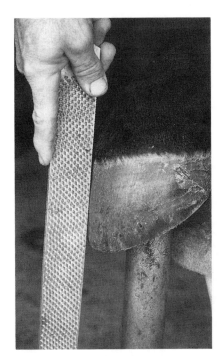

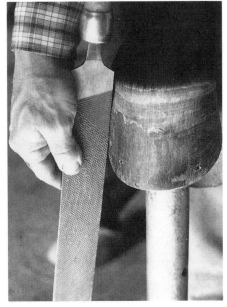

Checking for flare

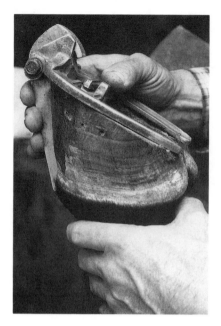

Measuring hoof angle

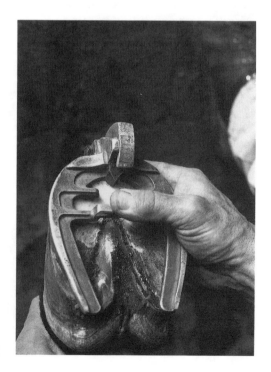

Reading the hoof gauge

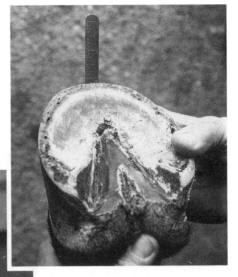

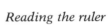

Measuring toe length

Reading the ruler

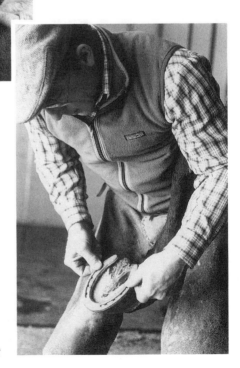

Checking shoe fit

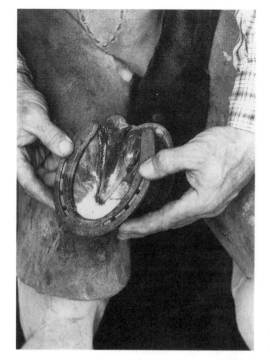

Positioning the shoe on the hoof

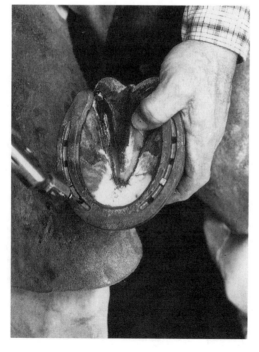

Nailing

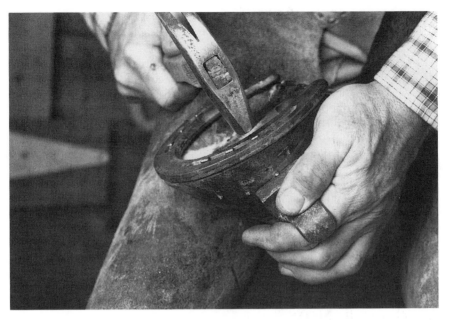

Setting clinches

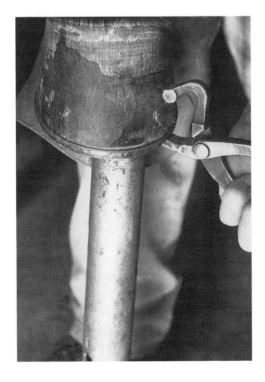

Clinching

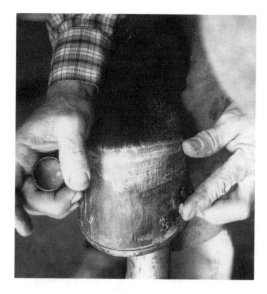

Filling nail holes

RESET OR NEW?

The decision of whether to reset shoes or use new ones is best left to your farrier. Generally, if the branches of the shoe are wearing evenly, the shoes can be reset until there is no longer a deep enough crease remaining to protect the nail heads. Another limiting factor is the wear on the hoof surface of the shoe from expansion (Chapter 5). Sometimes grooves are worn so deeply that there is no longer a flat surface for the freshly trimmed hoof. Also, if optimum traction is critical for a performance, new shoes may be required.

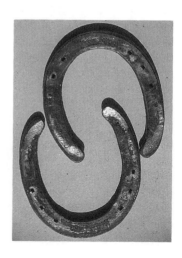

Grooves from heel movement

Amount of shoe wear is affected by the type of shoe (size, thickness, material), how much the horse is used, how the horse uses his hooves (e.g., does he drag his toes?), how much the horse self-exercises and in what manner, and the type of footing the horse travels over. Some horses will wear out a set of steel shoes in five weeks, with very little riding time, because of the way they exercise. Horses with vices such as weaving, pacing or pawing have unique and usually accelerated shoe wear patterns. Certain horses' shoes might show so little wear that the same shoes can be reset four or five times. The wear (rounding) a shoe receives at the toe is usually beneficial to a horse's movement and is one advantage to resetting. Bar shoes often last longer than open shoes because of the added amount of shoe surface taking the wear.

More often than not, a shoe will have to be reshaped, however slightly, before it is reset onto the trimmed hoof. When reforming a long-toed, low-heeled hoof, for example, it is common for the hoof to become rounder and shorter over consecutive shoeing periods. Most farriers charge the same for a reset as for new shoes because the time required to clean and reshape the shoes for reset is the same or more than the time to prepare new shoes.

SHOEING QUALITY CONTROL CHECKLIST

Hoof Preparation

Static vs. dynamic balance • Toe-heel tubule alignment • Dorsal-palmar (plantar) balance • Medial-lateral balance • Length • Levelness • Sole • Frog • Shape • Symmetry of hoof pairs

Shoe Preparation

Selection • Fit • Hoof expansion • Heel support • Contact with the wall • Sole pressure

Nails

Heads • Placement • Pattern • Clinches

Details

HOOF PREPARATION

Static vs. Dynamic Balance *Static balance* refers to a geometric equilibrium of the hoof when it is at rest. Generally when the ground surface of the hoof is perpendicular to the axis of the limb (when viewed from the front, the medial and lateral walls are equal in length and the coronet is parallel to the ground), the hoof is in static balance. *Dynamic balance* takes into account the action of the hoof and limb. In its most complete sense, dynamic balance refers to the relationship of all the limbs in motion. In order for a hoof to be functionally balanced for efficient motion and symmetric strides, the trimming and shoeing must take conformation and other factors into consideration (Chapter 8). Achieving dynamic balance, especially when working on a gait abnormality, often involves trial and error. While static balance addresses appearance, dynamic balance focuses on function. The more hoof and limb conformation deviate from standard guidelines, the less likely static and dynamic trimming techniques will produce similar results.

Toe-Heel Tubule Alignment The angle of the hoof at the heel should be parallel to the angle at the toe. When the heel angle is 5 degrees less

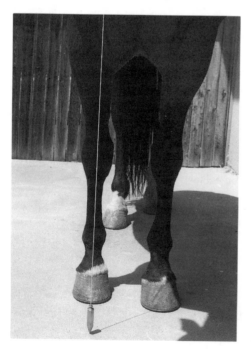

Balance assessment

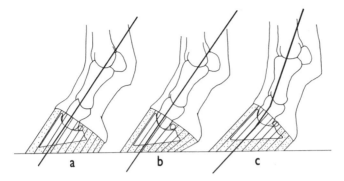

a. Normal: tubules parallel from toe to heel
b. Underrun heel: tubules not parallel
c. Low heels: tubules parallel

than the toe angle, the hoof is said to have underrun heels. In such a case, the horn tubules at the heel are crushed and collapsed forward and are often more nearly parallel than perpendicular to the ground surface. It is as if the tubules at the heel are "lying down on the job." Rarely is the heel angle steeper than the toe angle, but it may appear that way if the toe is allowed to grow out with a dish.

Dorsal-Palmar (DP) Balance DP balance refers to the hoof angle (relationship between the dorsal wall of the hoof and the ground) and the alignment of the hoof angle and the pastern angle. Hoof angle is measured at the toe with a hoof protractor. For years textbooks cited 45 to 50 degrees as a "normal" front hoof angle and 50 to 55 for hinds. But everyday observations by practicing farriers and recent research indicate that normal front pastern and hoof angles for domestic riding horses range from 53 to 58 degrees and normal hind angles from 55 to 60 degrees, with the odd normal horse outside of these ranges. (The range of toe angles in wild horses has been reported to be 50 to 60 degrees in the front and 53 to 63 degrees in the hind.)

Each horse has his own "ideal" hoof angle. The angle of the hoof is considered correct when the hoof and pastern are in alignment, that is, the dorsal surface of the hoof is parallel to an imaginary line (axis) passing through the center of the long pastern bone. The goal is actually to align the dorsal surface of the coffin bone with the long pastern bone axis. The hoof wall is used as a guide, since in the normal hoof the dorsal surfaces of the hoof wall and coffin bone are parallel.

This alignment is best viewed from the side of the horse, with the horse standing squarely on a hard, level surface with the cannon

The pastern angle is represented by a line through the center of the long pastern bone, not a line at the dorsal surface of the pastern.

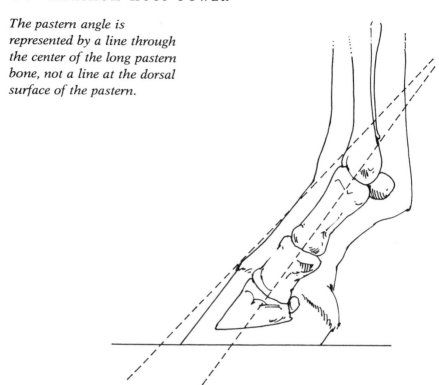

bones vertical. It is important to use a line through the center of the long pastern bone for the pastern angle. Using the irregular surface formed by hair and skin at the front of the pastern will result in inaccurate alignment.

Since more lamenesses are associated with low heels (and low hoof angle) than steep heels (and higher hoof angles), and since the hoof angle gets progressively lower during the five to eight-week shoeing cycle (because the toe grows faster than the heel), it is usually best for the horse to be shod a little on the steep side.

If the hoof angle is too low in relation to the pastern angle, the center line will be broken back near the vicinity of the coronary band. The more a hoof angle is lowered, the more the pastern angle raises and the more broken back the hoof-pastern axis becomes. Decreasing hoof angle increases the strain on the deep digital flexor tendon.

If the hoof angle is too high in relation to the pastern angle, the line will be broken forward. The more a hoof angle is raised, the lower the pastern angle becomes and the more broken forward the hoof-pastern axis becomes. Increasing hoof angle decreases the strain on the deep digital flexor tendon but does not change the strain on the superficial flexor tendon or suspensory ligament.

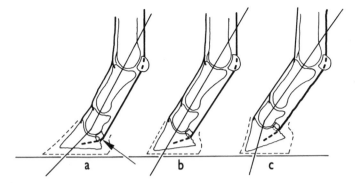

a. Broken back axis
b. Straight axis (Note: It is normal for the bottom of the coffin bone to be 5 to 7 degrees above the horizontal.)
c. Broken forward axis Richard Klimesh drawing

Medial-Lateral (ML) Balance ML balance refers to the relationship between the medial (inside) wall of the hoof and the lateral (outside) wall of the hoof. Determining ML balance is one of the most challenging aspects of farriery and relies as much on art as it does on science. The goal is to trim the hoof in such a way that the ground surface of the hoof is centered beneath the limb. This will allow the hoof structure to bear the weight of the limb evenly. Altering the relative lengths of the sides of the hoof will shift the position of the hoof beneath the limb. Lowering the lateral wall tends to position the hoof more toward the midline of the horse, while lowering the medial wall will tend to position the hoof away from the midline of the horse. But repositioning the limb by trimming may have undesirable consequences.

There are many methods for determining ML balance, none of which will work for all horses. Whether a farrier (or veterinarian) chooses a static or dynamic approach and which specific guideline he follows depends on his experience, the age of the horse, the degree of abnormality and the accompanying problems.

One method of achieving *static* ML balance is to trim the hoof so the coronet is parallel to level ground. This works with relatively straight limbs. But if a hoof has remodeled over a period of years to accommodate deviations in the limb, this trimming method may put uneven stress on the limb.

A similar method is to trim the hoof so that the plane of the ground surface is perpendicular to the cannon bone. A "T-bar" or similar device can be used to make this determination. This method is also suitable for normally conformed limbs.

Another method is to trim the hoof so that its ground surface is perpendicular to the midline of the horse. This can be checked by picking up the forelimb. With the horse's knee flexed and the cannon lightly resting in the hand, site across the ground surface of the hoof. This approach works well on horses having limbs that deviate from the ideal and will often result in *dynamic* ML balance.

It is generally agreed that the hoof is in dynamic balance when the medial and lateral walls strike the ground at the same time. If a hoof is landing on the lateral wall first, that side is assumed to be longer and should be trimmed shorter to allow a flat landing. If a horse *lands* on its lateral toe, it often *loads* on its medial heel. This diagonal imbalance can cause a jamming up of the coronary band at the medial heel, which can result in sheared heels (Chapter 11).

Some horses are so conformed that it is impossible to achieve a flat landing. Overzealous trimming should be avoided, for lameness could result from attempting to make a sound horse's apparently unbalanced hooves conform to an "ideal." It is important to realize that the way the hoof contacts the ground differs with each gait. A hoof that does not land flat at the walk may land flat at the trot or canter. Landing flat is only one guideline to balance, not a hard and fast rule.

Many hooves, especially hinds, cannot be balanced dynamically by trimming the medial and lateral sides of the hoof to be equal in length. Examining the shoe for wear can help determine a plan for trimming that will result in even wear on both branches of the shoe. Usually, if the side of the hoof that shows the least amount of shoe wear is trimmed shorter, the subsequent wear on the shoe will be equal. This rule is excepted by a horse that is lame or has an unusual

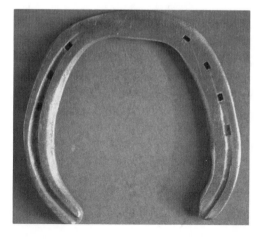

Uneven shoe wear: the crease is completely worn away on one branch.

way of going, so it is wise not to rely on just one guideline when attempting something as complex as balancing the equine limb. When using the above method (or any method), it is very valuable to record the trimming approach and to label and save the used shoes so that changes in the wear pattern can be noted and future trimming adjusted accordingly.

If the hoof wall is worn too short to balance by trimming alone, wedge pads, shims or custom shoes can be used to achieve balance until the hoof grows.

Length The length of the hoof is measured at the center of the toe from the point where the soft coronet meets the hard hoof wall (coronary rim) to the ground surface (see photograph on page 37). The toe length determines the length of the lever that the limb must break or pivot over. Long toes create a longer lever arm, a delayed breakover and increased pressure on the palmar/plantar portions of the distal limb. However, trimming the toe too short can invite bruises.

The appropriate toe length of a freshly trimmed hoof ready for shoeing will vary according to a horse's hoof conformation and breed. For example, the toe length of a small Arabian might be 3 inches, a Quarter Horse 3½ inches and a warmblood 4 inches. If a horse is to be barefoot, the hoof is left ¼ inch longer than if the horse is to be shod. The optimum length of the hoof wall is actually dictated by the optimum thickness of the sole.

Levelness The entire bottom of the hoof wall should be level so it makes perfect contact with a smooth ground surface or a flat shoe. Any unevenness will cause the hoof to bear weight unevenly. In some cases, however, a farrier may purposely remove a portion of the hoof wall at the ground surface to "relieve" a crack, flare or displaced coronet (Chapter 11). In most instances, however, the hoof wall should be level.

Sole The natural sole is slightly cupped from side to side as well as from front to rear. At time of trimming, your farrier will pare the sole to a concave shape but not so thinly as to cause the horse to be sore when he walks on gravel. If the sole is left too thick, however, it reduces hoof expansion during weight bearing and may inhibit the natural springing action of the hoof capsule, which is an important shock-absorbing function. Also, a thick sole will often prevent the farrier from trimming the toe sufficiently to attain DP balance. The bars should not be weakened by excessive trimming, but long, deformed horn should be removed.

Frog The frog should be smoothly pared, with no loose or overgrown tissue that could trap dirt and manure and harbor anaerobic thrush organisms. The clefts of the frog at the heels should be trimmed out so that the hoof can self-clean. It is not necessary or desirable for the frog to bear weight when the horse stands on level ground.

Shape The inside wall is generally steeper than the outside wall. The wall at the toe is usually thicker than at the quarters. The entire hoof wall from the coronary band to the ground should be straight, that is, without dips or bulges. Flares and dishes tend to be self-perpetuating. If there are any dishes (dips in the toe) or flares (dips in the sides of the hoof), the wall should be rasped straight. This will encourage the growth of a normal hoof shape (Chapter 11).

To evaluate shape, find the normal center of the sole, most recently referred to as Duckett's Dot. On the *average riding* horse, Duckett's Dot is located ⅜ inch back from the tip of the trimmed frog. Once the horse's hoof has been trimmed and shaped, the distance from the Dot to the toe should equal that from the Dot to the outermost border of the medial wall. The distance from the Dot to the lateral wall is usually greater.

Symmetry of Hoof Pairs Generally, the toe length of a hoof should be equal to that of its mate. However, variation in hoof angle often occurs in paired limbs due to individual limb conformation. In some instances, the difference should be minimized through trimming and shoeing, but in many cases the mismatched limbs should be allowed to be different. Dynamic balance will indicate which path the farrier chooses. In some cases the hooves will be trimmed and shod differently so that they move the same (Chapter 11).

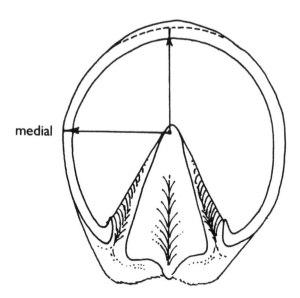

Duckett's Dot

There is a normal difference in shape and hoof angle between fore feet and hind feet. Most fore feet are larger, rounder and wider at the heels and have a flatter sole than the same horse's hind feet. Hind feet are commonly one shoe size smaller and more pointed at the toe and have a more concave sole and higher hoof angle.

SHOE PREPARATION

Selection The size of the shoe should be appropriate for the size of the horse and hoof. The shoe should be strong enough to support the horse's weight but not unnecessarily heavy or it might negatively affect the horse's stride and agility. The shoes should provide adequate protection, support and traction. The nail heads are protected from wear by setting them in either a crease or a hole stamped in the shoe.

Hot vs. cold shoeing can refer to the way the farrier makes, shapes and/or applies shoes. Hot shoeing can mean the farrier makes the shoes from scratch in a forge or modifies keg shoes in a forge or fits a hot shoe to the hoof. Cold shoeing means the farrier shapes and applies the shoe without heating it up. Many farriers use a combination of hot and cold shoeing techniques.

Fit A shoe should follow the natural shape of the properly prepared hoof, being neither too wide nor too narrow, too short nor too long. When viewed from above with the foot on the ground, from $\frac{1}{16}$ to $\frac{1}{8}$ inch of the edge of the properly fitted shoe will be visible from the quarters back to the heels. This indicates that the shoe has adequate allowance for heel growth and expansion.

Hoof Expansion A shoe is fit full to accommodate heel movement and normal increase in hoof width during the five- to eight-week shoeing period. With each step, as the horse's weight descends on the foot, it causes movement (expansion) at the heels. As the weight is lifted, prior to breakover, the heels return (contract) to their original position. These events are evidenced by the grooves worn in the hoof surface of the shoe. Ask your farrier to show them to you the next time he removes one of your horse's shoes (see photograph on page 40).

Because the hoof is cone-shaped, as it grows longer the base of the cone essentially gets wider, while the steel shoe that is nailed to it remains its original size. That's why it is necessary to start out with the shoe wider, so that after three to four weeks there is still support for the heel area of the hoof, which is now wider than when the shoe was applied.

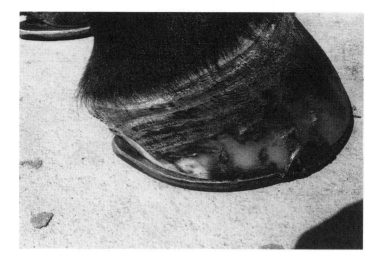

Good shoe fit

Too little expansion room will allow the hoof wall to spread over the edge of the shoe as it grows, resulting in lack of support and hoof wall damage. Too much expansion room increases the chance that the horse will step on the shoe or catch it on something. Upright hooves need less expansion room than flatter, spread-out hooves with more sloping walls.

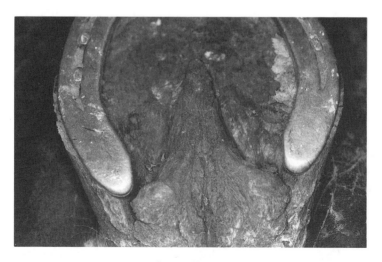

Hoof spread over shoe

Heel Support Enough shoe should extend beyond the heels so that the limb is adequately supported. Generally the heel of the shoe should be below the midline of the cannon bone when the cannon is vertical. Another guide is that the length of the shoe is equal to or greater than twice the toe length of the prepared hoof. "Short shoeing" (using a shoe that is too small) does not provide ample support, can result in fatigue and permanent damage to the horse's limbs and lead to underrun heels.

Contact with the Wall Unless some of the hoof wall is missing from hoof damage or has been purposely removed to treat a crack or a persistent flare or other abnormality, the shoe should contact the hoof wall completely. The corner of a business card should not fit between the hoof and the shoe at any point around the outside perimeter of the hoof. Hot-fitting a shoe properly (heating the shoe and pressing it onto the prepared hoof) provides a perfect match between shoe and hoof. When a shoe is cold fit, the farrier must be skilled with a hammer and rasp to be sure the hoof and shoe meet all the way around.

Sole Pressure Although the shoe should be in contact with the entire hoof wall, it should not contact more than ⅛ inch of the sole. If a horse has very flat soles, the inner edge of the hoof surface of his shoes will need to be relieved to avoid creating unwanted sole pressure (see also figure on page 32). This is especially important when the horse is shod with wide-web shoes. Sole pressure can disrupt blood flow and lead to lameness, abscesses and corns.

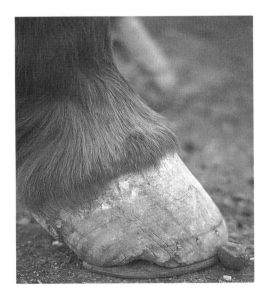

Short shod

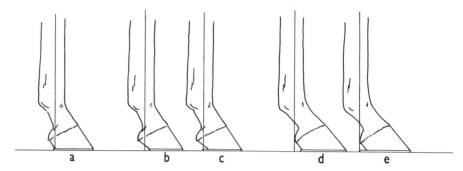

Heel Support

a. An ideal situation: the hoof is in DP balance, the heels are not underrun and there is proper heel support. In this case, shoes that extend just slightly behind the heels of the hoof provide adequate support.

b. Although this hoof is in DP balance, the toe-heel alignment is not parallel and the heels are underrun. When the shoe is fit to the heels, the hoof is "short shod" and inadequately supported.

c. The same hoof as in B, but properly supported with a longer shoe.

d. This hoof is in DP balance and the toe-heel alignment is parallel, but the low hoof-pastern angle results in the hoof being too far ahead of the limb. When the shoe is fit to the heels, the hoof is "short shod" and inadequately supported.

e. The same hoof as in D, but properly supported with a longer shoe. Richard Klimesh drawing

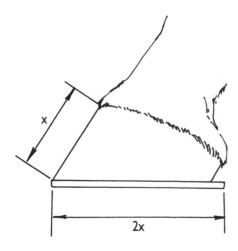

A shoe length guide

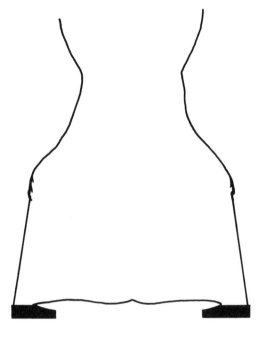

The hoof surface of the shoe is relieved to prevent sole pressure

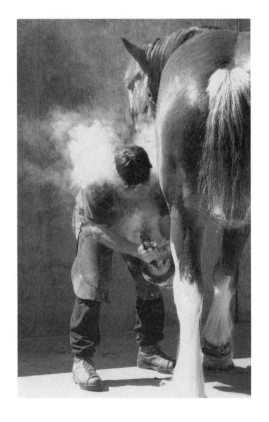

Hot-fitting a shoe

NAILS

Heads The nail head should seat tightly in the crease or stamped hole and should protrude below the shoe about 1/16 inch.

Placement The nail should enter the hoof within the white line. If the nail enters outside the white line, the clinches will likely be too low and the shoe may not be secure. If the nail enters inside the white line, sensitive structures will probably be invaded (Chapter 11). The tip of the nail is beveled so that it travels in a curved path in dense horn tissue and exits the hoof wall. If the nail is angled to the center of the hoof or placed inside the white line, the soft tissue there may not provide enough resistance to curve the nail outward, and the nail will not exit the hoof wall. The bevel is on the same side as the pattern on the nail head. The nail is placed with the bevel toward the inside of the hoof, so when driven the nail will curve away from the bevel. Six to eight nails are used, generally none placed behind the widest portion of the hoof wall. The heel nail holes on most keg shoes are often located too far rearward, so only six nails are used, leaving the heel nail holes empty.

Pattern The height of the nail farthest back on the shoe should be approximately one third the distance from the ground to the coronary band. The nail pattern is affected by the quality of the hoof, the skill of the farrier and the quality and design of the shoes and nails

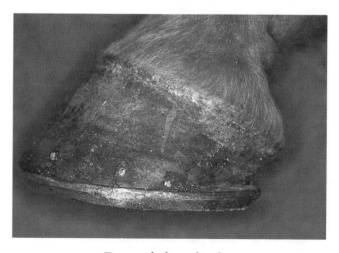

Extremely low clinches

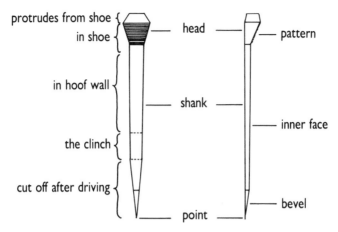

Parts of a nail. Richard
Klimesh drawing

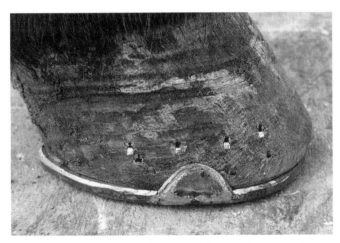

*Clinches showing good size, height, and pattern. Note
the nail holes have not yet been filled. Also note
squared-toe shoe.*

being used. Ideally, the nail pattern should form a straight line and
the two toe nails should be at equal heights when viewed from the
front.

Clinches The clinches should be "square," that is, only as long as
they are wide. Such clinches will open easily, allowing the shoe to
come off if it gets caught on something. Rectangular clinches are

longer than they are wide. Since such clinches usually hold the shoe on very securely, if a horse gets the shoe caught on a fence or steps on it, he may rip large portions of his hoof off along with the nails and the shoe (see photograph on page 229). Clinches should be uniform and set flush with the hoof wall, and should not be set into a groove filed in the hoof wall. They should feel smooth when you run your hand over them (see photograph above).

DETAILS

The hoof wall should be smooth, never rasped above the clinches unless necessary to remove a flare. The edge of the hoof wall as well as the edge of the shoe should be smooth. Old nail holes should be filled with a wax (see Resource Guide in the Appendix) or other appropriate substance to prevent moisture, mud and other contaminants from entering the hoof.

Any exposed edges of the shoe should be rounded (see figure on page 32) with a rasp or grinder to decrease the chance that the shoe will come off if stepped on. Also, this removes any burrs or steel slivers that may injure a person handling the feet.

If the Shoe Fits...

Steel, the material most commonly used in making horseshoes, is a combination of iron and other elements, mainly carbon. Steel is graded by the amount of carbon it contains; the higher the carbon content, the harder the steel. Mild (low-carbon) steel is used for horseshoes because it is easily shaped and yet durable enough to last for one or more shoeing periods. A high-carbon steel, such as used for springs or tools, would last longer but would be more difficult to shape and would have less traction on hard surfaces. All but the largest sizes of mild steel horseshoes can be shaped while cold to fit the hoof. Large shoes, as for warmbloods and draft horses, must be heated in a forge to be shaped.

OTHER SHOE MATERIALS

Aluminum is lighter than steel. Because of this weight advantage, most racing shoes, or "plates," are made of aluminum. A shoe made of aluminum can be made wider for support or thicker to alter DP balance without the weight increase associated with a similar steel shoe. Because it's softer than steel, however, aluminum does not wear as well, and many aluminum shoes are equipped with steel inserts at the toes, where the most wear occurs. Modern manufacturing processes are producing shoes of aluminum alloys that wear much longer than the earlier aluminum shoes. However, if these shoes are heated for shaping or forming clips, the wear is often greatly reduced.

Aluminum shoes bend or spring more easily than steel shoes,

which means they often cannot provide the support that a horse needs. This is especially true with larger horses or with jumpers, where there is a great deal of force upon landing and turning.

Another drawback of aluminum horseshoes is that in the presence of moisture, galvanic corrosion occurs between the steel nails and the aluminum. This reaction corrodes the hoof surface of the shoe and affects the hoof itself. Evidence of this corrosion is seen as a pasty white substance between the shoe and hoof when the shoe is removed.

Titanium is a corrosion-resistant element having the strength of steel and the lightness of aluminum. Because it was considered a strategic material until recent years, civilian access to and research with titanium have been limited. Testing is underway that may result in a titanium shoe that can be worked like a conventional shoe and that will provide the best properties of both steel and aluminum.

Attempts have been made for years to develop a successful plastic horseshoe. The main drawback to nail-on plastic shoes is that the inherent flexibility of the material does not provide sufficient support for a horse's hoof. Also, the slippery surface of the plastic encourages the hoof to spread over the edges of the shoe.

Plastic horseshoes that are glued to the hoof wall by means of a cuff or series of tabs are very valuable in therapeutic applications (see photograph on page 162). They are used when the wall is too damaged or weak to securely hold nails and on foal hooves that are too thin walled to safely nail. Since application of glue-on shoes is relatively nontraumatic, they are often used on laminitic horses and other horses in extreme pain.

There are several types of horseshoes available that combine a core of steel or aluminum with an outer shell of plastic or rubber. These shoes give more support to the hoof than plastic alone, and many can be shaped like a conventional steel shoe. The "advantage" of these shoes is their ability to absorb shock. Yet there is a scarcity of independent research concerning the effectiveness of shock-absorbing hoof wear and on the effects of shock on the equine limb.

SHOE TYPES

Horseshoes are either individually hand-forged by the farrier or they are mass-produced in a factory. At one time factory-made shoes were transported in wooden kegs, so the term *keg shoe* refers to a ready-made commercial shoe. When keg shoes were lacking in both quality

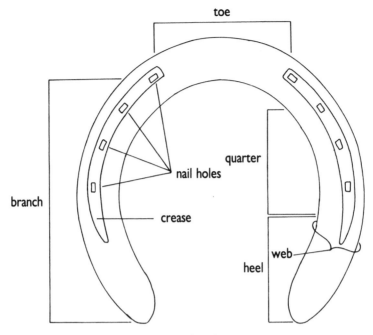

Parts of a shoe

and variety, it was worth the farrier's time to hand-forge the shoes he used. Today keg shoes are available in many shapes, materials, thicknesses, widths and qualities. Many top farriers seldom find it necessary to make a shoe from bar stock, while others enjoy the forge work so much that they hand-make all the shoes they apply.

It is very common for farriers to modify keg shoes to suit particular purposes. The most common modifications are repositioning the nail holes, adding a bar, altering the shape of the toe (rolled, rocker, square), altering the heel shape and length (trailers, extended heels, spooned heels) and forging or attaching clips.

The most common types of keg shoes used on riding horses are the plain shoe, the rim shoe and the half-round shoe (see photograph above). Breed and performance organizations often have specific shoe regulations described in competition rules.

Bar Shoes

A bar can be placed anywhere across the branches of a shoe to stabilize the shoe, protect the hoof from ground contact and trauma and provide added support. The type of bar shoe used will vary according to the need. A straight bar connects the heels of the shoe and protects the frog. If the frog is very prominent or the heels very low, the bar can be set away from the frog and is called a drop bar. A cross bar can go diagonally or straight across the shoe at any location to protect the sole or the navicular area of the frog.

A myth concerning bar shoes is that they cause contracted heels. In fact, a properly applied bar shoe will *encourage* hoof expansion. Any type of shoe will contribute to heel contraction if the nails or clips are placed so far back as to restrict hoof movement (Chapters 5 and 11).

It is imperative that a bar that crosses the hoof does not contact the sole at any point, since it could impair circulation within the foot or cause bruises and abscesses. When using a bar to protect the hoof, it is important to keep debris (bedding, manure, rocks, dirt, etc.) from accumulating, since this will put pressure on the sole during weight bearing and defeat the purpose of the bar. A full pad with careful attention to amount of packing may be helpful. When a pad is used for protection with a cross bar, it must be riveted to the bar to hold the pad away from the sole.

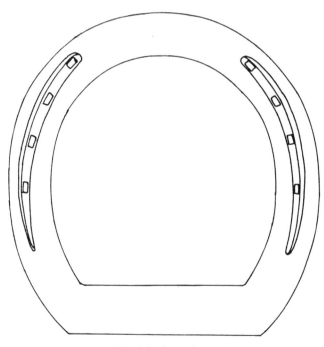

Straight bar shoe

SHOE CLUES

Materials

Steel • Aluminum • Titanium • Plastic • Plastic or rubber over a steel or aluminum core

Types

Plain shoe   a flat shoe having a crease (also called a fuller or swedge) on the ground surface of the shoe in the area of the nail heads.

Stamped shoe   a flat shoe without a crease, but with pockets stamped in the shoe for the nail heads; also called a punched shoe.

Rim shoe   a shoe with a crease around the entire ground surface for traction and for recessing the nail heads.

Training plate   a light, thin steel shoe.

Polo shoe   a light, thin steel rim shoe with a higher inside rim; stronger than a training plate.

Barrel racing shoe   a light, thin steel rim shoe with a higher outside rim.

Toed and heeled   a steel shoe having a bar protruding across the ground surface of the toe and a square protrusion called a calk at each heel to provide traction in soft footing.

Half-round   a shoe with stamped nail holes that is flat on the hoof surface and round on the ground surface.

Racing plate   a very light, thin aluminum shoe usually with a steel wear insert at the toe; available in a wide variety of styles.

Wedge shoe (swelled heel)   a steel or aluminum shoe thicker at the heel than at the toe.

Wide-web shoe   a shoe formed from wider steel (see page 62, lower photo).

Sizes

There is no standard among horse shoe companies regarding shoe sizes. A shoe that has a 14-inch circumference (from heel to heel) could be one of eight different sizes (ranging from #1 to #12), depending on the company that makes it. The Farrier Industry Association has developed a chart that categorizes most available steel, aluminum and plastic horse shoes according to their circumference from heel to heel (see Resource Guide in the Appendix).

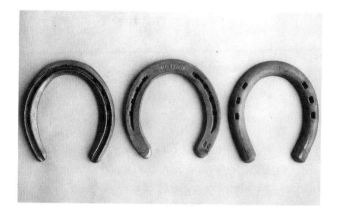

From left: Rim shoe, plain shoe, half-round shoe

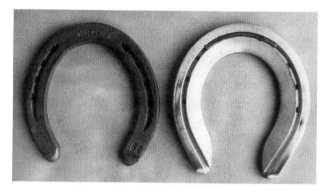

From left: Plain steel shoe, wide-web aluminum shoe

Egg Bar Shoe A shoe with extended branches that curve inward and connect to each other at the heels is an egg bar. Egg bar shoes provide a large, stable base which extends behind the heels. This longer base supports the heels in soft footing, prevents the hoof from rocking back and takes some stress off the deep digital flexor tendon and the navicular area.

Egg bar shoes can often interrupt the undesirable cycle leading to contracted heels, collapsed, underrun heels and flat soles. A flat-soled hoof is a "dead hoof," one that lands with a thud; it is not conformed

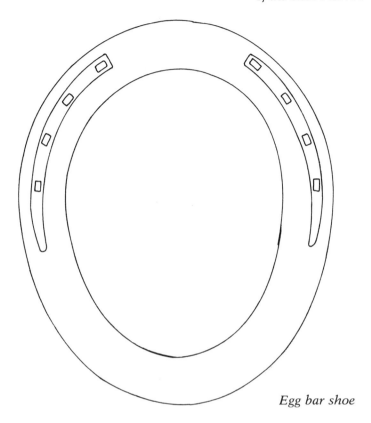

Egg bar shoe

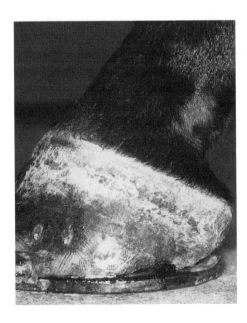

Egg bar shoe

TYPES OF SHOES AND DEVICES THAT AFFECT TRACTION

Standard keg shoe   Plain steel shoes, whether creased or punched, usually provide adequate traction for most situations.

Aluminum shoes   Aluminum shoes have a slightly better grab than steel shoes because aluminum is softer. Aluminum racing plates with toe grabs and/or heel stickers can be used successfully in some situations.

Rim shoes   Rim shoes provide added traction because the rims, until they are worn down, cut into the ground. Also, the dirt that packs into the swedge provides more traction against the ground than does a flat steel shoe.

Toed and heeled shoes   In winter conditions, such as semifrozen ground or "soft" ice, these shoes will give good traction. On hard ice or rocks, however, they are less effective than rim shoes.

Borium   (tungsten carbide) or other hard surfacing materials can be applied to the ground surface of the horse's normal shoe in smears, beads or points on the toe and/or heels (see photograph on page 25; see Resource Guide in the Appendix).

Nails   Commercial frost or mud nails with ribbed or specially hardened heads can be substituted for regular horseshoe nails to provide added traction. One at each midpoint nail position may be all that is necessary. The treated and/or pointed heads resist wear and dig into hard ground or ice.

Calks   Calks are projections added to the ground surface of the shoe for providing traction. They can be permanent or removable (Chapters 4 and 10; see Resource Guide in the Appendix).

to transmit resilient energy. Such a hoof shod with an egg bar shoe may, over time, begin to develop a more cupped (concave) sole, a desirable configuration that encourages a trampoline-like contraction and expansion resulting in the hoof springing off the ground.

By virtue of the shape of the bar and the extra amount of material in an egg bar shoe, the horse's weight is spread out over a larger area of ground than with a conventional shoe. An egg bar shoe instantly gives a horse a larger base of support. This is particularly important for horses that have a disproportionate relationship between their body weight and the circumference of their hooves (heavy horses, small hooves).

The egg bar shoe is especially beneficial for the Thoroughbred-type hoof with heels that have collapsed forward and inward, resulting in an underrun hoof, often with a flat sole. It is equally helpful for the warmblood-type hoof, which is often flared outward on the sides with heels collapsed forward. When factors cause the tubules to begin angling forward, the hoof can quickly get caught in a self-perpetuating chronic condition that is often irreversible (Chapter 11).

The weight of a horse with underrun heels or a long toe/low heel axis is concentrated at the back of the hoof or even *behind* the hoof, causing excess tendon stress. In soft or deep footing, the larger ground surface of an egg bar "catches" the horse's weight as it descends down the limb, thereby reducing the strain on the deep flexor tendon and relieving some of the tension on the navicular region and the coffin joint. The egg bar extends the base of support and effectively redirects the horse's weight forward toward the center of the hoof. This will contribute to the development of a more desirable, upright hoof/pastern axis.

Because the bar of an egg bar is located behind the frog, the heel bulbs are protected. The egg bar shoe not only prevents the heels from sinking down into soft footings but protects the bulbs from the destructive trauma of striking the ground.

The hoof must be trimmed properly before an egg bar shoe is applied. If the toe is left long, it will impede breakover and defeat the purpose of the shoe. Modifying the toe of the shoe can ease breakover. The egg bar shoe should be fitted wide from the broadest part of the foot toward the rear. The length of the egg bar shoe will depend on

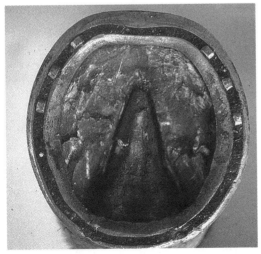

Squared-toe egg bar shoe

the configuration of the hoof. It may be so short as to resemble a straight bar shoe or it may extend to the back of the heel bulbs, forming a true egg shape.

Because the egg bar shoe consists of more material than a standard shoe, the action of the horse may be affected by the additional weight. The hoof may reach a higher arc in its flight, and the knees and hocks may exhibit a greater degree of flexion. During extension, the slight increase in weight at the end of the limb may result in a slight exaggeration of the horse "throwing the foot forward." If this is the case and the action is undesirable, an aluminum egg bar is appropriate.

Depending on the circumstances, the horse wearing bar shoes may require different management. A bar shoe tends to collect and retain bedding, mud or manure, so the hooves must be cleaned regularly. Horses wearing egg bars should not be turned out in deep or muddy footing.

The egg bar shoe is used in a wide variety of therapeutic applications, ranging from sheared heels to chronic suspensory problems. Egg bar shoes are also used on performing show jumpers; hunters; dressage, cutting and reining horses; pleasure and trail horses. In addition to increasing the useful life of a horse, the egg bar shoe encourages the development of a more correct and functionally sound hoof. Recognition of the value of egg bar shoes has prompted several manufacturers to add both steel and aluminum egg bar shoes to their product lines.

Heart Bar Shoe This shoe is basically a straight bar shoe with a specialized frog plate. In treating laminitis, the heart bar shoe is used to support the coffin bone. Since the heart bar is not used on performance horses, it will not be discussed in detail. (See Recommended Reading in the Appendix.)

Full Support Shoes A full support shoe is an egg bar shoe with a frog support plate. Steel and aluminum full support shoes are available commercially or can be made by a qualified farrier. (They are sometimes incorrectly called heart bar/egg bar because the shoes look similar.)

The full support shoe is used to treat hooves with flat or dropped soles and hooves with very weak and/or underrun heels. A portion of the horse's weight is carried by the frog plate, allowing the heels of the hoof to grow down without being crushed. Some performance horse owners prefer to continue using these shoes even after the hooves have attained a satisfactory condition.

This shoe is also very useful in the treatment of hooves that have had a portion of the hoof wall removed (as in a heel resection for a crack) or injured (as in a heal tear). Contrasted to an egg bar shoe,

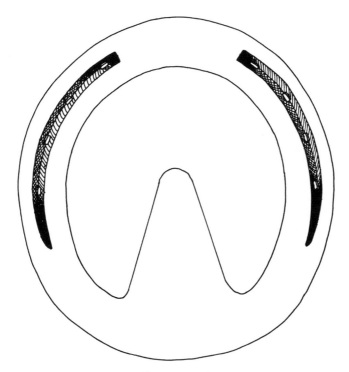

Full support shoe

which is used to support a hoof that has had the heel "floated" to allow a displaced heel to descend to the shoe, the full support shoe is used when it is desirable to stabilize the hoof capsule while the hoof grows new horn.

A full support shoe is fit in the same manner as the egg bar shoe described above. The frog plate should follow the shape of the frog and support it completely from ½ inch back from the tip of the trimmed frog. When the shoe is set on the prepared hoof, the entire frog plate should just contact the frog, not apply pressure. The frog support plate should not extend beyond the boundaries of the frog or circulation within the hoof might be impaired. If the frog is recessed from the level of the hoof wall, shims of the appropriate size and shape can be attached to the frog plate to achieve contact.

The configuration of the full support shoe makes it difficult to keep the sole clean, especially if the horse is in mud, gravel or dirty bedding. If the hoof wall is of poor quality or the horse is in undesirable footing, a full pad may need to be used with the full support shoe.

In lieu of a full support shoe, a full support pad can be used. This type of pad also is available commercially or can be fabricated by an experienced farrier. It is difficult to properly fit the pad to the frog, however, since the opaque pad surface prevents direct observation of frog contact. To function properly, the ground surface of the pad must be supported beneath the frog either by a frog plate on the shoe or by the addition of a frog-shaped shim (the thickness of the shoe) on the pad itself.

Extended Heel Shoes

Extended heel shoes are used to lengthen the base of support for the limb. In an ideally conformed hoof, the amount of shoe extended past the heel of the hoof will be from ⅛ to ¼ inch, enough to allow for the normal forward migration of the shoe over the five- to eight-week shoeing period. Hooves with varying degrees of underrun heels will require more length of shoe to achieve the necessary support.

The branches of extended heel shoes, when applied to the front feet, usually curl inward (often approximating the shape of an egg bar shoe), and in fact they are often called open egg bars. On the hind feet, the heels can be bent straight back to form a true extended heel shoe or bent outward 45 degrees to form bilateral trailers. Bilateral trailers widen as well as lengthen the support base, adding stability to the limb. Also, with the shoe heels bent backward or outward, the clefts of the frog clean easier than with an open egg bar shoe.

The danger of using trailers or "straight-back" extended heel shoes on the fronts is that the heels of the shoe are very likely to be stepped on by the hinds. Halters should never be left on loose horses, but leaving one on a horse that wears extended heels is likely to result in a devastating accident. Extended heel shoes are an excellent preventive shoe and performance enhancer when used on horses engaged in strenuous athletic activities such as dressage and jumping.

Wide-Web Shoes

Wide-web shoes are used to protect the perimeter of the sole and to provide more ground contact and a more stable support for the hoof. They have gained popularity with the increase in the population of the larger warmblood horses. Because of their extra width, these shoes are more resistant to deforming under the weight of a horse. Also, their increased surface area is thought to dissipate some of the shock of impact.

One drawback to an increase in the area of ground surface contact by the shoe is a decrease in traction. Therefore, when used on per-

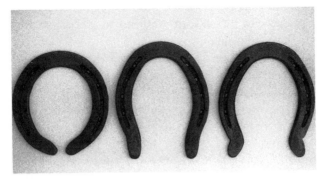

From left:
open egg bar, extended heels, bilateral trailers

formance horses, wide-web shoes often require some sort of traction device (Chapters 4 and 10). The inner edge of the ground surface of the wide-web shoe can be made concave with a hammer or grinder to increase traction (see figure on page 32).

When a wide-web shoe is used on a hoof with a flat sole, it is necessary to relieve or seat (see figure on page 32) the inner edge of the hoof surface of the shoe or apply a rim pad between the shoe and the hoof wall to prevent pressure on the sole. On some commercial wide-web shoes, the nail holes are placed proportionately farther inward on the web. This might be fine for a thick-walled hoof, but when these shoes are used on a thin-walled hoof, the farrier has to be very careful to avoid driving a close or hot nail. This is less of a problem with hand-forged wide-web shoes because the farrier can take the horse's hoof wall thickness into account when he makes the nail holes in the shoe.

Other Types of Shoes

Treatment Plate A treatment plate, or hospital plate, is used to protect the sole or frog and is designed to allow relatively easy access to these areas for daily inspection and medication. A treatment plate is used in cases of dropped sole, protruding coffin bones, sole abscesses and puncture wounds to the sole or frog. Although a hard plastic pad or metal plate can simply be taped to the bottom of a shoe to serve the same purpose, if treatment is expected to extend for more than a few days, a treatment plate that bolts on to the bottom of the shoe will be much more economical in terms of both time and money. Treatment plates can be custom made by an experienced farrier and are available commercially.

Contiguous Clip Shoe The Contiguous Clip Shoe (designed by Richard Klimesh) is used in treating fractures of the coffin bone, an injury associated with barrel horses, roping horses, jumpers and other horses that turn sharply at speed. The shoe is made by fitting a straight bar or egg bar shoe closely to the hoof, with no allowance for normal expansion. (The purpose of this shoe is to *prevent* movement of the hoof capsule while the fractured bone heals.) Often a rocker or squared toe is used to minimize the pull of the deep digital flexor tendon on the coffin bone during breakover. Approximately six to eight tall clips are welded around the outer perimeter of the shoe. After the shoe is nailed on, a fast-setting acrylic material is applied between the hoof and clips, essentially encasing the lower half of the hoof in a cast (see Resource Guide in the Appendix).

Modified Toe Shoes

Various modifications to the toe of a shoe can decrease the force needed for breakover and shorten the time the hoof is on the ground (Chapters 7 and 9).

Squared Toe The toe of the shoe is squared or made straight across and set back from the toe of the hoof to facilitate easy breakover. The toe of the hoof is usually rounded with the rasp to prevent chipping. Used on the hinds, squared-toe shoes will help prevent the stepping off of front shoes.

Roller Toe The hoof surface of the shoe is flat. The ground surface of the shoe has a rounded toe much like a naturally worn shoe.

Rocker Toe Half the web of the toe of the shoe is bent upward. This requires that the toe of the hoof be rasped or cut to fit the shoe. The hoof is encouraged to break over specifically at the point of the rocker location.

Roller-Motion Shoe Combining the rocker toe with swelled heels results in a roller-motion shoe.

Half-Round Shoe The ground surface of the outside and inside edge of the entire shoe are round. A half-round shoe allows a horse to break over more easily in any direction.

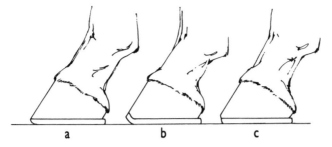

Modified toe shoes
a. Rolled toe
b. Rocker toe
c. Squared toe

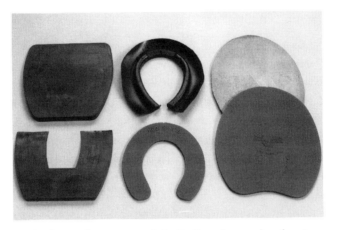

Clockwise from upper left: Full wedge pad, tube rim pad, full leather pad, full plastic pad, rim pad, bar wedge pad

PADS

There are four main reasons to use hoof pads: to change the angle of the hoof, to protect the hoof, to reduce concussion and to prevent snowballing.

A full pad covers the entire bottom of the horse's foot and is installed between the hoof and the shoe with or without hoof packing.

TYPES OF PADS

Full flat pads   Pads in leather, plastic or metal that cover the entire sole. They are used to protect the sole and to keep it clean.

Leather pads compress between the shoe and the hoof and conform to the sole. They absorb water and will deteriorate. They can allow more normal hoof respiration than plastic pads.

Plastic pads are available in a variety of thicknesses, hardnesses, colors, and durability that allow many types to be reset. They do not allow the hoof to respire and may or may not conform to sole.

Metal pads are made of thin steel or aluminum, provide positive protection to the sole and frog and greatly reduce traction.

Shock absorbing pads   Pads intended to reduce concussion and vibration to the hoof and limb structures.

Wedge pads   Tapered pieces or wedges of material, usually plastic, placed between the shoe and the hoof. They are generally used to raise the heels of low-heeled hooves. When placed sideways, a wedge pad can be used to alter the ML balance by making the short side of the hoof taller. Wedge pads are also called degree pads because they are manufactured in various thicknesses or degrees. They are available as a full pad or bar pad. A bar pad is solid across the thick end and open in the middle. Thicker wedge pads are often stiff enough across the heels to protect the frog and underlying navicular area from direct ground pressure.

Bubble Pads   Full, hard plastic pads with 2-inch diameter domes molded into the center of the ground surface. Originally designed for anti-snowballing, they can also be used to relieve pressure over the navicular region or another sole area. With bubble pads, traction is reduced and a thick shoe is required to prevent the bubble from bearing the horse's weight.

Rim Pads   These fit between the shoe and the hoof wall; the sole and frog are open. They are used to put more distance between the sole and the ground.

Tube Type Rim Pads   This type of pad is comprised of a small rubber tube that lines the inside rim of the shoe and is held in place by an attached flat, thin tab (flange), which lies between the shoe and the hoof. They are designed to eliminate snowballing.

Full pads are made of leather, metal, plastic or other synthetic materials. Side clips (discussed later in this chapter) are often used with pads to help maintain the position of the pad and shoe on the hoof and to decrease the shearing stress on the nails.

Horses that have inherited the genetic formula for flat and/or thin soles may benefit from wearing full pads. Even horses that have a normally concave sole, if worked on gravel or rocky terrain, may require full pads to prevent bruising.

Along with the use of full pads, though, comes an interruption in the balance of hoof respiration. As hooves "breathe" they release moisture. You can see evidence of this if your horse is barefoot or shod without pads and is standing on a rubber mat. When you pick up his foot you will likely see a circular patch of hoof fog on the mat. When a full pad covers the sole of a hoof, this outward moisture migration is halted, the moisture collects under the pad, and the hoof structures can become softened and weakened. In addition, full pads tend to trap invading slush, mud and snow, which provide a suitable environment for growth of bacteria, fungus and yeast. Some farriers believe that horses develop an even thinner and more vulnerable sole from wearing pads full time and therefore become "pad dependent." However, it has been observed that some horses with weak soles develop a thick normal sole with the use of full pads and *proper* hoof packing.

Traction is decreased with a full flat pad; the cup of the bare sole and the frog are covered, therefore the only traction provided is from the grip of the shoe. Full support pads have an artificial frog built onto the ground surface, and a new hydroplastic pad conforms completely to the contours of the frog and sole. Both of these pads help compensate for traction loss. The added weight of a pad and packing can exaggerate a horse's action and travel deviations.

There are many pads on the market that claim to protect the horse by reducing concussion. Although research has recently shown there *is* a difference in the shock-absorbing capacity of various pads, exactly which pads are effective and how effective they are is undocumented and widely debated. A properly shod healthy foot provides all the shock absorption necessary for normal work by transferring the energy of the hoof's impact to the shock-absorbing structures: hoof wall, laminae, frog, digital cushion and blood vessels. If the hoof structures are abnormal or the work is excessive, concussion-reducing pads are sometimes prescribed. Success will depend on the type of pad used, the amount and type of packing, the horse's conformation and degree of soundness, the footing and other management factors.

A wide variety of concussion-reducing pads are available as full pads or rim pads. The material of the pads must have the ability to absorb the force of concussion quickly and release it slowly. Because of the repeated compression and expansion of the pad, the pad may become permanently compressed, permanently spread out or actually cut through by the hoof wall. The result may be loose clinches, premature wearing of the nail holes, loose or lost shoes and possible weakened or split hoof walls.

For a discussion of anti-snowballing pads, see Chapter 10.

Some breed and performance associations have rules specifically related to the use of hoof pads at horse competitions. It is the horse owner's and exhibitor's responsibility to know and abide by any regulations related to shoes or pads.

Hoof Packing

There are differing opinions on whether to pack the space between the pad and the hoof and what materials to use for packing. Although tradition calls for pine tar with oakum, using it has drawbacks. Oakum is a loose, stringy hemp fiber that retains water, disintegrates and shifts beneath the pad, often working out between the heels. The most recent popular option is silicone caulking, which is either squirted into the sole space from a caulking gun after the shoe and pad are in place or mixed with a catalyst to speed curing and applied to the sole before the shoe and pad are nailed on. There are several significant drawbacks to using silicone, however. It tends to concentrate moisture and heat against the sole, and if too large an amount is used, it puts pressure on the sole and prevents the sole from descending as part of its normal shock-absorbing function. Also, silicone allows sand and mud to accumulate between the pad and the sole, causing sole pressure.

Commercial hoof-packing preparations can be used with varying degrees of success (see Resource Guide in the Appendix).

CVP Method A healthy alternative for packing is the CVP Gasket Pad, developed by Richard Klimesh. *CVP* stands for the three main ingredients: copper sulfate powder, venice turpentine, and polypropylene hoof felt. Poly felt, which does not readily absorb water, was developed specifically as a hoof-packing material. Copper sulfate is a salt used in agriculture to control fungi, bacteria and yeast. Venice turpentine is a thick resin from the larch tree. The copper sulfate and venice turpentine combine to make a medicated adhesive that binds the poly felt to the sole, forming a gasket between the pad and the hoof. This gasket protects the hoof wall and sole from the invasion of sand, dirt, mud, water, and other foreign matter for the entire five- to eight-week shoeing period. It eliminates the foul odor often associated with the use of other packing. The CVP packing forms a barrier against the hoof that prevents excess moisture from baths, creeks or muddy pens from softening the hoof and helps to restore weak or damaged hooves. Often when a horse loses a shoe, the CVP will still adhere to the sole. (See Resource Guide in the Appendix.)

CLIPS

A clip is a vertical extension of a horseshoe that is used to secure shoes on horses with poor-quality hooves, to help restore and retain hoof shape, to take the shear stress off the nails on very active horses, and in the construction of various therapeutic shoes. To balance the forces exerted on the clips, they are normally applied symmetrically in opposing pairs.

Weak, shelly hoof walls that have difficulty holding nails are candidates for clips. If the hoof wall is pithy or brittle, using a clip on each side of the shoe may help keep the shoe on while new horn replaces the poor-quality hoof. Side clips are commonly installed either between the first and second or second and third nail holes from the toe. These clip locations prevent the shoe from moving back on the hoof or to either side. However, technique and skill allow a farrier to use clips anywhere on the shoe that they are required.

Flares at the quarters can often be contained by proper rasping and the addition of quarter clips, usually between the third and fourth nail holes of a factory shoe (Chapter 11).

For low to moderately active horses, six nails will usually hold a shoe on a healthy, high-quality hoof for six to eight weeks. However, when an active horse speeds up, slows down, turns, jumps or stops hard, his shoes are subjected to twisting and sliding forces that can cause the nails to loosen and the shoe to shift on the hoof or be lost. Horses that have traction devices such as calks or borium on their shoes always can use the added security that clips provide.

Sometimes a horse might strike the ground toe first, causing the shoe to shift rearward on the hoof. This can occur on the fronts of hunters and jumpers from the impact of landing, on the hinds of reining horses from hard stops, on the hinds of many types of horses as they unload from trailers and on any hoof from kicking a wall or stomping at flies. To help keep the shoe from being forced back, a single clip can be added at the toe.

Care must be taken that a toe clip does not hold the shoe out ahead

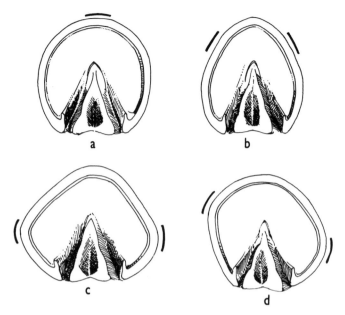

Clip positions
a. Toe clip
c. Rearward-placed side clips
b. Forward-placed side clips
d. Asymmetric side clips

of the hoof wall. This would move the base of support too far forward and impede breakover. For this reason, many farriers prefer to use a pair of forward-placed side clips rather than a single toe clip. Also, if a modified toe shoe is used, a toe clip is impractical, if not impossible to apply.

In the treatment of some injuries or lamenesses, clips may be helpful. For example, in the case of hoof cracks, expansion may be undesirable. With each step, a crack may open and spread upward. Properly placed clips minimize hoof movement. If a portion of hoof wall is removed (resected), limiting the area in which to nail, clips will help secure the shoe until the wall is replaced (Chapter 11).

Your farrier might forge or draw clips from a hot shoe or weld or braze clips onto the shoe. The base of a clip should be a little wider than the web of a normal shoe, or about 1 inch. The height of the clip should be as wide as the web of the shoe, or about ½ inch to ¾ inch and higher if a pad is used. The thickness at the base should be about 1/16 inch. The clip tapers from the base to the tip and the point should not be sharp but well rounded and thin, so that if the shoe comes off and the horse steps on the clip, it will bend over and not puncture his hoof. The clip should incline inward, parallel to the hoof wall.

Clips are often drawn, hammered to the desired angle and then seated into position on the hoof while the shoe is still hot. Because of the angle of the clips, it is difficult to hot-fit some rearward-placed quarter clips, especially if they are designed to contain flares. In those cases, when the clips are formed, the angle is left a bit more open than the angle of the hoof wall. This allows the base of the drawn quarter clips to be seated hot into the hoof. After the shoe is nailed on, the upper portion of the clip is tapped toward the hoof to conform to the slope of the hoof wall. Instead of hot fitting, some farriers carve or file out a notch in the hoof wall where the base of the clip will seat.

Drawn clips are limited in height and width by the amount of steel that can be pulled from the hot shoe. When a pad is used between the shoe and hoof, only the very tip of a drawn clip may extend high enough to contact the hoof wall. Clips that are brazed or welded on can be of any height or width and have an advantage not only with pads but in cases where the clip needs to extend past a void in the hoof wall to contact solid horn.

NAILS

You might think that all horseshoe nails are the same, but there are many different sizes, types and qualities of nails available. The nail that your farrier chooses can make a significant difference in the quality of the shoeing job. When a shoe is applied, the heads of the nails should fit tightly into the crease and protrude about 1/16 inch below the shoe. If the size and shape of the nail head is not appropriate for the shoe, the nails can shear or loosen, resulting in loose and lost shoes.

A nail with a thick, wide shank displaces too much hoof material and can cause a hoof to split and crack. The slimmest nail that will secure the shoe should be used.

The type of steel, the design, and the finish on the nail will determine how easily and accurately it can be driven into the hoof wall. This is very important, since the nails are driven within millimeters of sensitive tissues and often must be strategically placed to avoid old nail holes, cracks and voids in the hoof.

A hard nail will be more difficult to clinch, but the clinch will hold more securely. A soft nail will be easy to clinch and will also open up more readily. If your horse steps on his shoe or catches it in a fence, it is better if the clinches open up and allow the nails to slip through the hole in the hoof rather than for the clinches to hold very tightly and rip off large portions of hoof (see photograph on page 229).

Movement and Performance

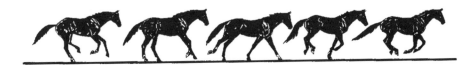

C H A P T E R   7

Freeze Frame

Evaluation of movement and performance requires a certain base of knowledge and a "good eye." To develop your ability to "see" rather than just "look," you need to be able to periodically stop the action in your mind's-eye camera so you can analyze the various components of a movement. In this chapter we're going to push the pause button and then use single-frame advance to analyze the natural gaits of the horse and the phases of the stride. Once you get a fix on the components of a movement, you will have a better chance of analyzing the motion in real time.

To further assist the development of your eye, study horse performances on video. When you view videotapes, be sure they are properly tracked in your VCR. If your VCR has at least four heads you can use stop action, single-frame advance and slow motion features.

Filming your own horse's movement can provide you with a valuable visual analysis of gait, movement abnormalities and responses to various shoeing modifications. A videotape is a permanent record that you can view repeatedly and use as reference when reevaluating a movement problem. When videos are played in slow motion, you can determine at what precise time a particular limb deviation occurs. When the frame is "frozen," it will even allow you to take photographs of the image on the screen or to measure particular components on the screen.

With the rapid advances in video technology, portable equipment is affordable and easy to operate. In order to get the best-quality image, a camcorder (portable video camera/recorder) with a high-speed shutter (1/500 minimum for walking and trotting and 1/1000 for faster work) should be used. Recording with fast shutter speed will give a sharper image when the tape is played at slow motion, freeze-frame and single-frame advance.

THE NATURAL GAITS

Walk The walk is a four-beat gait that should have a very even rhythm as the feet land and take off in the following sequence: left hind, left front, right hind, right front. A horse that is rushing at the walk might either jig or prance (impure "gaits" comprised of half walking, half trotting), or he might develop a pacey walk. The pace is a two-beat lateral gait where the two right limbs rise and land alternately with the two left limbs. Although the pace is a natural gait for some Standardbred horses and other breeds, a pacey walk is considered an impure gait for most riding horses because the even four-beat pattern of the walk has been broken.

Trot The trot is a two-beat diagonal gait. Traditionally, trot refers to an English gait with moderate to great impulsion. The (western) jog is a shorter-strided trot with less impulsion. The right front and left hind rise and fall together alternately with the diagonal pair left front and right hind. Often the trot is a horse's steadiest and most rhythmic gait. If a horse is jogged too slow, the gait becomes impure, as the diagonal pairs break and the horse essentially walks behind and trots in front.

Canter The canter or lope is a three-beat gait with the following sequence: one hind limb, then the other hind limb and its diagonal forelimb, and finally the remaining forelimb. If a horse is on the right lead, the initiating hind (sometimes referred to as the driving hind) will be the left hind, the diagonal pair will be the right hind (sometimes referred to as the supporting hind) and the left front, and the final beat will occur when the leading foreleg, the right front, lands. Then there is a moment of suspension as the horse gathers his limbs underneath himself to get organized for the next cycle. (A change of lead should occur during the moment of suspension so the horse can change front and hind simultaneously.) When observing a horse on the right lead from the side, you can observe that the right limbs reach farther forward than the left limbs.

Gallop The gallop or run is a four-beat accelerated variation of the canter. With increased impulsion and length of stride, the diagonal pair breaks, resulting in four beats. The footfall sequence of a right lead gallop is left hind, right hind, left front and right front. As in canter, the right limbs will reach farther forward than the left limbs

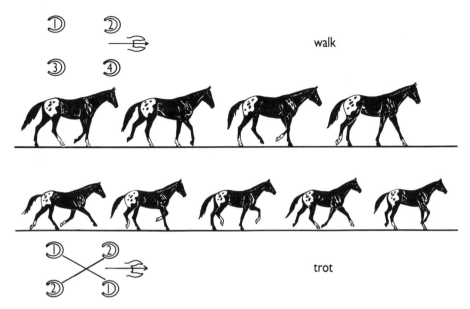

walk

trot

The walk and trot. From *From the Center of the Ring* by Cherry Hill, Garden Way Publishing

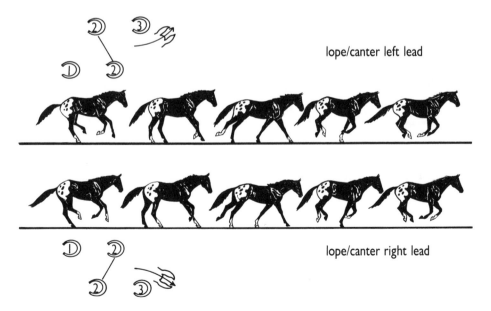

lope/canter left lead

lope/canter right lead

The canter/lope, left lead and right leads. From *From the Center of the Ring* by Cherry Hill, Garden Way Publishing

when the horse is in the right lead. There is a more marked suspension at the gallop than the canter.

Back The back, performed in its correct form, is a two-beat diagonal gait in reverse. The left hind and right front are lifted and placed down together, alternating with the right hind and left front.

THE PHASES OF A STRIDE

The phases of a horse's stride are landing, loading, stance, breakover and swing.

Landing The hoof touches the ground, the limb begins to receive the impact of the body's weight.

Loading The body moves forward and the horse's center of gravity passes over the hoof. Usually this is when the fetlock descends to its lowest point, sometimes resulting in an almost horizontal pastern. The cannon is vertical.

Stance The fetlock rises to a configuration comparable to the horse's stance at rest. The transition between the loading phase and the stance phase is very stressful to the internal structures of the hoof and lower limb. The horse's center of gravity moves ahead of the hoof. The flexor muscles and tendons lift the weight of the horse (and rider) and the fetlock begins to move upward. The pastern straightens and the limb begins pushing up off the ground.

Breakover Breakover is the phase when the hoof prepares to leave the ground. It starts when the heels lift and the hoof begins to pivot at the toe. At that moment the knee (or hock) relaxes and begins to flex. Breakover is measured from the time the heels lift to the time the toe leaves the ground. The deep digital flexor tendon (assisted by the suspensory ligament) is still stretched just prior to the beginning of breakover to counteract the downward pressure of the weight of the horse's body.

Swing The limb moves through the air and straightens out in preparation for landing.

STRIDE LENGTH

For years it was believed that leaving the toe of a hoof long would increase a horse's stride length, thereby contributing to a smooth and efficient stride and less strides over a given distance. In the past, race

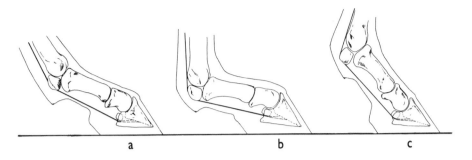

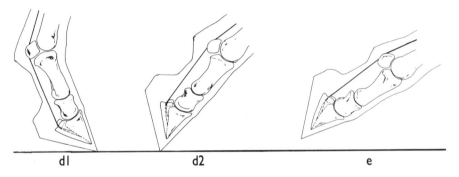

The phases of the stride

a. Landing
b. Loading
c. Stance

d1. Breakover—heel lift
d2. Breakover—toe pivot, just prior to toe lift
e. Swing

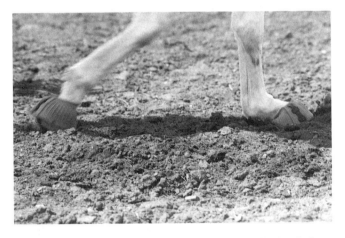

One limb at mid-breakover and one fully loaded

horses, show ring hunters, jumpers and even Western Pleasure and reining horses have been shod with long toes and low heels to supposedly create a performance advantage. Research has shown that contrary to popular opinion, horses with long toes and an acute hoof angle do not take longer strides.

Long toes (often accompanied by low, underrun heels) put the pivot point of the hoof farther forward than normal. The long toe acts as a lever arm as the hoof moves from the loading phase to the stance phase and attempts to break over. The long toe makes it more difficult for the heels to rotate around the toe, consequently tension in the deep digital flexor tendon may be prolonged and/or exaggerated. Additionally, the navicular ligaments, which stabilize the navicular bone and which are already stretched to the maximum at the beginning of breakover in a normal hoof, are stressed excessively during the breakover of a hoof with a low angle (see figure on page 85). The delayed breakover causes the mass of the horse's body to move farther forward over the horse's limbs before the limbs leave the ground.

Recent research has shown that the arc of hoof flight is not significantly changed by trimming. However, the approach to the loading phase and the landing phase is affected. With a normally trimmed hoof, the toe of the hoof elevates slightly prior to landing as the hoof prepares for a heel-first or flat-foot impact. The hoof with an acute angle approaches the ground toe first, often landing with the toe impacting first. Such stabbing into the ground with the toes can result in a broken, jarring motion (and sometimes stumbling) rather than smooth action.

During the trot, when the fronts are trimmed normally and the hind toes are long, the hinds leave the ground significantly later than their diagonal forefeet. However, the hind limbs compensate for the delay in breakover by moving through the air more rapidly so they can land at the same time as their corresponding diagonal forefeet. This causes an unevenness in the gait; the hind limbs are initially delayed and then hurry to catch up.

The research also disproves the popular theory that long toes on the hind may make a horse reach farther forward. On the contrary, rather than the hind limbs reaching farther forward, the horse's mass moves further ahead of the weight-bearing limbs before they leave the ground. This tends to put the cycle of the forelimb movement further under the horse, thereby lessening the potential for (hindquarter) engagement and putting extreme pressure on the navicular area of the front limbs.

Talk the Movement Talk When talking about your horse's movement with your farrier, veterinarian or trainer, it helps if you all use correct, descriptive terms. Rather than saying, "This horse isn't moving well," far more information is transmitted by saying, "At the trot, my horse's *stride* is shortened and *uneven* and his *rhythm* is *irregular*."

TERMS ASSOCIATED WITH MOVEMENT

Action The style of the movement, including joint flexion, stride length and suspension; usually viewed from the side.

Asymmetry A difference between two body parts or an alteration in the synchronization of a gait; when a horse is performing asymmetrically, he is often said to be "off."

Balance The harmonious, precise, coordinated form of a horse's movement as reflected by equal distribution of weight from left to right and an appropriate amount of weight carried by the hindquarters.

Breakover The moment between the stance and swing phases as the heel lifts and the hoof pivots over the toe.

Cadence See rhythm.

Collection A shortening of stride within a gait, without a decrease in tempo; brought about by a shift of the center of gravity rearward; usually accompanied by an overall body elevation and an increase in joint flexion.

Directness Trueness of travel, the straightness of the line in which the hoof (limb) is carried forward.

Evenness Balance, symmetry and synchronization of the steps within a gait in terms of weight-bearing and timing.

Extension A lengthening of stride within a gait, without an increase in tempo, brought about by a driving force from behind and a reaching in front; usually accompanied by a horizontal floating called suspension.

Gait An orderly footfall pattern such as the walk, trot, canter.

Height The degree of elevation of arc of the stride, viewed from the side.

Impulsion Thrust, the manner in which the horse's weight is settled and released from the supporting structures of the limb in the act of carrying the horse forward.

Overtrack   Or "tracking up"; the horse's hind feet step on or ahead of the front prints.

Pace   The variations within the gaits such as working trot, extended trot, collected trot; a goal (in dressage) is that the tempos should remain the same for the various paces within a gait. Also refers to a specific two-beat lateral gait exhibited by some Standardbreds and other horses.

Power   Propelling, balancing (and sometimes pulling) forces.

Rapidity   Promptness, quickness, the time consumed in taking a single stride.

Regularity   The cadence, the rhythmical precision with which each stride is taken in turn.

Relaxation   Absence of excess muscular tension.

Rhythm   The cadence of the footfall within a gait taking into account timing (number of beats) and accent.

Sprain   Injury to a ligament when a joint is carried through an abnormal range of motion.

Step   A single beat of a gait. A step may involve one or more limbs. In the walk there are four individual steps. In the trot there are two steps, each involving two limbs.

Stiffness   Inability (re: pain or lack of condition) or unwillingness (re: bad attitude) to flex and extend the muscles or joints.

Strain   Injury (usually to muscle and/or tendon) from overuse or improper use of one's strength.

Stride, length of   The distance from the point of breaking over to the point of next contact with the ground of the same hoof; a full sequence of steps in a particular gait.

Suppleness   Flexibility.

Suspension   The horizontal floating that occurs when a limb is extended and the body continues moving forward; also refers to the moment at the canter and gallop when all limbs are flexed or curled up, reorganizing for the next stride.

Tempo   The rate of movement, the rate of stride repetition; a faster tempo results in more strides per minute.

Travel   The path of the hoof (limb) flight in relation to the midline of the horse and the other limbs; usually viewed from the front or rear.

Factors That Affect Movement and Performance

Many elements work synergistically to produce movement. When movement is evaluated, traditionally lower limb conformation, lameness and shoeing are the focal points of the analysis. However, many other factors can cause subtle to dramatic alterations in a horse's movement.

CONFORMATION AND TYPE

While movement is most evident in the lower limbs, it is an integration of the action of the upper limbs, back, neck, in fact, the whole horse. Therefore, overall conformation must be considered when discussing movement. For sake of completeness, a thorough conformation analysis follows. Certain conformation tends to lead to certain types of movement. However, there are no absolutes when it comes to predicting a horse's length of stride, degree of flexion or directness of travel. Generalizations related to stance, breed or type are peppered with exceptions.

Conformation refers to the physical appearance of a horse as dictated primarily by his bone and muscle structures and his outline. It is impractical to set a single standard of perfection or to specifically define *ideal* or *normal* conformation because the guidelines depend on the classification, type, breed and intended use of a horse. A conformation evaluation should always relate to specific function.

When discrepancies are discovered, it is important to differentiate between blemishes and unsoundnesses. Blemishes are scars and ir-

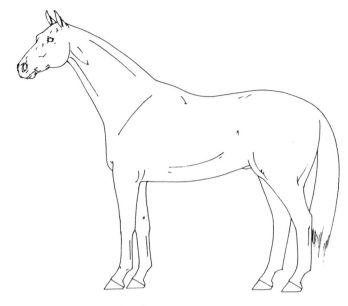

Conformation outline

regularities that do not affect the serviceability of the horse. Unsoundnesses cause a horse to be lame or otherwise unserviceable. Old
wire cuts, small muscle atrophies and white spots from old injuries
are considered blemishes if they do not affect the horse's soundness.
Unsoundnesses include but are not limited to lameness caused from
such conditions as navicular syndrome, wounds, ringbone, sidebone,
spavin, thoroughpin, curb and bowed tendons.

Horses are classified as draft horses, light horses or ponies. Clas-
sifications are further divided by type according to overall body style
and conformation and the work for which best suited. Light (riding
and driving) horses can be described as one of six types: sport, stock,
hunter, pleasure, animated (show) and race.

The sport horse can be one of two types: a large, athletic horse
suited for one or all of the disciplines of eventing (dressage, cross-
country and jumping) and typified by the European warmblood
breeds, or a small, lean, tough horse suited for endurance events and
typified by the Arabian. Stock horses are well-muscled, agile, and
quick, suited to working cattle and are typified by the American Quarter Horse. Hunters move with a long, low (horizontal) stride, so are
suited to cross-country riding and negotiating hunter fences and are
typified by the American Thoroughbred. Pleasure horses have comfortable gaits, are well designed for ease of riding and are typified by
the smooth-moving individuals in any breed. The animated (show)

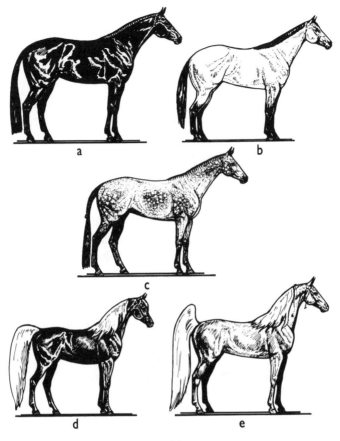

Types of horses

a. Sport horse (warmblood
type)
b. Stock horse
c. Hunter

d. Pleasure horse
e. Show horse From *From the
Center of the Ring* by Cherry Hill,
Garden Way Publishing

horse is one with highly cadenced, flashy gaits (usually with a high
degree of flexion) suited mainly for the show ring and is typified by
the American Saddlebred and some Morgans. The racehorse is lean in
relation to height with a deep but not round barrel and is typified by
the racing Thoroughbred.

A breed is a group of horses with common ancestry and usually
strong conformational similarities. In most cases, a horse must come
from approved breeding stock to be registered with a particular
breed. If a horse is not eligible for registration, it is considered a
grade or crossbred horse.

Several breeds can have similar makeup and be of the same type.

For example, most Quarter Horses, Paint Horses and Appaloosas are considered stock horse types. Some breeds contain individuals of different types within the breed. American Thoroughbreds can be of the race, hunter or sport horse type.

Making a Visual Assessment

Develop a specific system for evaluating horses. Be aware that wildly colored horses and those with dramatic leg markings can cause visual distortions that can result in inaccurate conclusions.

Begin by looking at a horse from the near side in profile and assess balance by comparing the forehand to the hindquarters. When viewing the horse in profile, pay attention to the curvature and proportions of the topline. Let your eyes travel from poll to tail and down to the gaskin. Then observe the manner in which the limbs attach to the body. Evaluate angles.

Step to the front of the horse and evaluate the limbs and hooves for straightness and symmetry. Observe the depth and length of the muscles in the forearm and chest. Evaluate the head, eyes, nostrils, ears and teeth.

Then step to the off side and confirm or modify your evaluation of the balance, topline and limb angles.

Move to the hindquarters and stand directly behind the tail. Evaluate the straightness and symmetry of the back, croup, point of hip and buttock and the limbs. Let your eyes run slowly from the poll to the tail, as this is the best vantage point for evaluating back muscling and (provided the horse is standing square) left-to-right symmetry. You may need to elevate your position if you are evaluating a tall horse. The spring of rib is also best observed from the rear view.

Now make another entire circle around the horse, this time stopping at each quadrant to look diagonally across the center of the horse. From your position at the rear of the horse, step to the left hind and look toward the right front. This angle will often reveal abnormalities in the limbs and hooves that were missed during the side, front and rear examinations. Proceed to the left front and look back toward the right hind. Move to the right front and look toward the left hind. Complete the revolution at the right hind looking toward the left front.

And finally, step to the near side and take in a view of the whole horse in profile once again.

While you are looking at a horse, it helps if you get an overall sense of the correctness of each of the four functional sections: the head/neck, the forehand, the barrel and the hindquarter.

Head and Neck The vital senses are located in the head, so it should be correct and functional. The neck acts as a lever to help regulate the horse's balance while moving. Therefore, it should be long and flexible, with a slight convex curve to its topline.

Forehand The front limbs support approximately 65% of the horse's body weight, so they must be strong and sound. The majority of lameness is associated with the front limbs.

Barrel The midsection houses the vital organs, therefore the horse must be adequate in the heart girth and have good spring to the ribs. The back should be well muscled and strong so the horse can carry the weight of the rider and the saddle.

Hindquarters The rearhand is the source of power and propulsion. The hindquarter muscling should be appropriate for the type, breed and use. The croup and points of the hip and buttock should be symmetric and the limbs should be straight and sound.

Conformation Components

Balance A well-balanced horse has a better chance of moving efficiently with less stress. Balance refers to the relationship between the forehand and hindquarters, between the limbs and the body and between the right and the left sides of the body.

The center of gravity is a theoretical point in the horse's body around which the mass of the horse is equally distributed. At a standstill, the center of gravity is the point of intersection of a vertical line dropped from the highest point of the withers and a line from the point of the shoulder to the point of the buttock. This usually is a spot behind the elbow and about two thirds the distance down from the topline of the back.

Although the center of gravity remains relatively constant when a well-balanced horse moves, most horses must learn to rebalance their weight (and that of the rider and tack) when ridden. In order to simply pick up a front foot to step forward, the horse must shift his weight rearward. How much the weight must shift to the hindquarters depends on the horse's conformation, the position of the rider, the gait, the degree of collection and the style of the performance. The more a horse collects, the more he steps under his center of gravity with his hind limbs.

If the forehand is proportionately larger than the hindquarters, especially if it is associated with a downhill topline, the horse's center of gravity tends to be forward. This causes the horse to travel heavy on his front feet, setting the stage for increased concussion, stress and lameness. When the forehand and hindquarters are balanced and the withers are level with or higher than the level of the croup, the horse's center of gravity is located more rearward. Such a horse can carry more weight with his hindquarters, thus move in balance and exhibit a lighter, freer motion with his forehand than the horse with withers lower than the croup.

When evaluating young horses, the growth spurts that result in a temporarily uneven topline should be taken into consideration. However, two-year-olds that show an extreme downhill configuration should be suspect. Even if a horse's topline is level, if he has an excessively heavily muscled forehand in comparison to his hindquarters, he is probably going to travel heavy on the forehand and have difficulty moving forward freely.

A balanced horse has approximately equal lower limb length and depth of body. The lower limb length (chest floor to the ground) should be equal to the distance from the chest floor to the top of the withers. Proportionately shorter lower limbs are associated with a choppy stride.

The horse's height or overall limb length (point of withers to ground) should approximate the length of the horse's body (the point of the shoulder to the point of buttock). A horse with a body a great deal longer than its height often experiences difficulty in synchronization and coordination of movement. A horse with limbs proportionately longer than the body may be predisposed to forging, overreaching and other gait defects (Chapter 9).

When viewing a horse overall, the right side of the horse should be symmetric to the left side.

Proportions and Curvature of the Topline The ratio of the topline's components, its curvature, the strength of loin, the sharpness of withers, the slope to the croup and the length of the underline in relation to the length of back all affect a horse's movement.

The neck is measured from the poll to the highest point of the withers. The back measurement is taken from the withers to the loin located above the last rib and in front of the pelvis. The hip length is measured from the loin to the point of buttock (see also figure above).

A neck that is shorter than the back tends to decrease a horse's overall flexibility and balance. A back that is very much longer than the neck tends to hollow. A very short hip, in relation to the neck or back, is associated with lack of propulsion and often a downhill configuration. A rule of thumb is that the neck should be greater than or equal to the back and that the hip should be at least two-thirds the length of the back (see figure on page 95).

The neck should have a graceful shape that rises up out of the withers, not dip downward in front of the withers. The shape of the neck is determined by the S shape formed by the seven cervical ver-

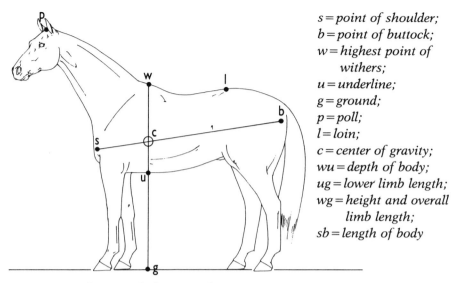

s = point of shoulder;
b = point of buttock;
w = highest point of
     withers;
u = underline;
g = ground;
p = poll;
l = loin;
c = center of gravity;
wu = depth of body;
ug = lower limb length;
wg = height and overall
      limb length;
sb = length of body

Center of gravity, balance, and proportion

tebrae. A longer, flatter (more horizontal) configuration to the upper vertebrae results in a smoother attachment at the poll *behind* the skull and results in a cleaner, more flexible throatlatch. If the upper vertebrae form a short, straight line to the skull, it is associated with an abrupt attachment *below* the skull, resulting in a thick throatlatch and possibly a hammerhead.

The curve to the lower neck vertebrae should be short and shallow and attach relatively high on the horse's chest. The thickest point in the neck is at the base of the lower curve. Ewe-necked horses often have necks that have a long, deep lower curve and attach low to the chest. The attachment of the neck to the shoulder should be smooth, without an abnormal dip in front of the shoulder blade.

The upper neck length (poll to withers) should be at least twice the lower neck length (throatlatch to chest). This is dictated to a large degree by the slope of the shoulder. A horse with a very steep shoulder has an undesirable ratio (approaching 1:1) between the upper neck length and lower neck length.

The back should look like it has a natural place for a saddle, beginning with prominent withers located above or behind the heart girth. The withers should gradually blend into the back, ideally ending at about the midpoint of the back. The withers provide a place for the neck muscles and ligamentum nuchae to anchor, and they should attach at the highest point of the withers. There should not be a dip in front of or behind the withers.

The withers also act as a fulcrum. As a horse lowers and extends

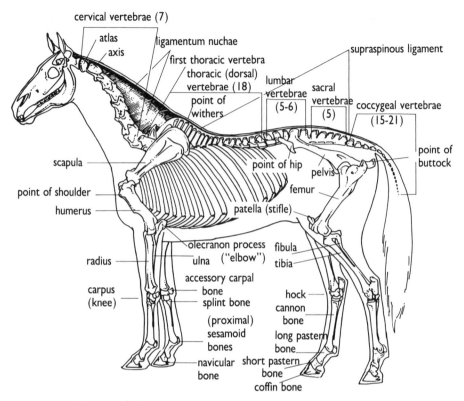

Equine skeleton. From *Making Not Breaking* by Cherry Hill,
Breakthrough Publishing

its neck, the back rises. Low, mutton withers limit a horse's ability to
raise his back. A horse with a well-sloped shoulder usually has correctly placed withers. The heart girth should be deep, which indicates adequate room for the heart and lungs.

The muscles that run alongside the spine should be flat and strong
rather than sloped or weak. The back muscles must help counteract
the gravitational pull from the weight of the horse's intestines as well
as to support the rider's weight.

The loin is located along the lumbar vertebrae from the last rib-
bearing (dorsal) vertebrae to the lumbosacral joint. The loin should
be well muscled and relatively short. Horses termed "long-backed"
often have an acceptable back length but a long, weak loin. A horse
with a weak and/or long loin and loose coupling tends to have a
hollow back. (The coupling is the area behind the last rib and in front
of a vertical line dropped from the point of hip.) A horse that chron-
ically hollows its back may be predisposed to back problems.

The loin and the coupling are what transfer the motion of the hindquarters up through the back and forward to the forehand, so they must be strong and well connected. A short, heavily muscled loin has great potential strength, power, and durability yet could lack the flexibility that a more moderately muscled loin may have. A lumpy appearance in the loin area may indicate partial dislocations of the vertebrae.

The croup is measured from the lumbosacral joint (approximately indicated by the peak above and slightly behind the points of hip) to the tail head. The croup should be fairly long, as this is associated with a good length to the hip and a desirable, forward-placed lumbosacral joint. The slope to the croup will depend on the breed and use.

The back should be "short" relative to the underline. Such a combination indicates strength plus desirable length of stride.

Head The head should be functionally sound. The brain coordinates the horse's movements, so adequate cranial space is necessary. The length from the ear to the eye should be at least one third the distance from ear to nostril. The width between the eyes should be a similar distance as that from the ear to the eye. A wide poll with ears far apart is associated with the atlas connecting behind the skull rather than below it. A wide-open throatlatch allows proper breathing during flexion; a narrow throatlatch is often associated with an ewe-neck attachment. Eyes set off to the side of the head allow the horse to have a panoramic view, and the eyes should be prominent without bulging. Prominence refers to the bony eye socket, not a protruding eyeball. The expression of the eyes should indicate a quiet, tractable temperament.

The muzzle can be trim, but if it is too small, the nostrils may be pinched and there may be inadequate space for the incisors, resulting in dental misalignments. The width of the cheek bones indicates the space for molars; adequate room is required for the sideways grinding of food. The shape of the nasal bone and forehead is largely a matter of breed and personal preference.

Quality Quality is depicted by "flat" bone (indicated by the cannon bone), clean joints, sharply defined (refined) features, smooth muscling, overall blending of parts and a fine, smooth haircoat. "Flat" bone is a misnomer because the cannon bone is round. Flat actually refers to well-defined tendons that stand out cleanly behind the cannon bone and give the impression the bone is "flat."

Substance Substance refers to thickness, depth and breadth of bone, muscle and other tissues. Muscle substance is described by type of muscle, thickness of muscle, length of muscles and position of attachment. Other substance factors include weight of the horse, height of the horse, size of the hoofs, depth of the heart girth and flank, and spring of rib.

Best viewed from the rear, spring of rib refers to the curve of the ribs; a flat-ribbed horse may have inadequate heart and lung space. Besides providing room for the heart, lungs and digestive tract, a well-sprung rib cage provides a natural, comfortable place for a rider's legs. A slab-sided horse with a shallow heart girth is difficult to sit properly; an extremely wide-barreled horse can be stressful to the rider's legs.

Substance of bone indicates adequacy of bone to weight ratio. Traditionally the measurement is taken around the cannon bone, just below the knee. For riding horses, an adequate ratio is approximately .7 inches of bone for every 100 pounds of body weight. Thus, a 1,200-pound horse should have an 8.4-inch cannon bone.

Correctness of Angles and Structures The correct alignment of the skeletal components provides the framework for muscular attachments. The length and slope to the shoulder, arm, forearm, croup, hip, stifle and pasterns should be moderate and work well together. There should be a straight alignment of bones and large clean joints when viewed from front and rear.

Forelimbs Both forelimbs should appear to be of equal length and size and to bear equal weight. A line dropped from the point of the shoulder to the ground should bisect the limb (see photograph on page 42). The toes should point forward and the feet should be as far apart on the ground as the limbs are at their origin in the chest. The shoulder should be well muscled without being heavy and coarse.

The muscles running along the inside and outside of the forearm should go all the way to the knee, ending in a gradual taper, rather than ending abruptly a few inches above the knee. It is generally felt that this will allow the horse to use its front limbs in a smooth, sweeping forward motion. The pectoral muscles at the horse's chest floor (an inverted V) should also reach far down on to the limb. These and the forearm muscles help a horse move its limbs laterally and medially as well as to elevate the forehand.

Limbs when viewed from the side should exhibit a composite of moderate angles, so that shock absorption will be efficient. The shoulder angle is measured along the spine of the scapula from the point of the shoulder to the point of the withers. The shorter and straighter the shoulder, the shorter and quicker the stride and the more stress and concussion transmitted to the limb. Also important is the angle the shoulder makes with the arm (which should be at least 90 degrees) and the angle of the pastern.

The length of the humerus (point of shoulder to the point of elbows) affects stride length. A long humerus is associated with a long reaching stride and good lateral ability; a short humerus, with a short choppy stride and poor lateral ability. The steeper the angle of

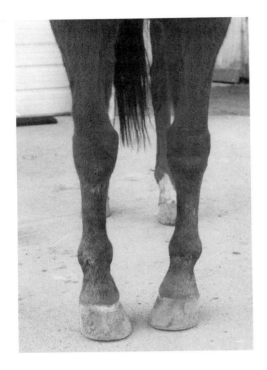

Toed in

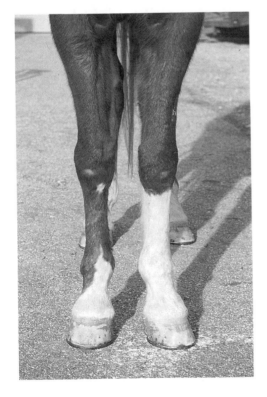

Toed out

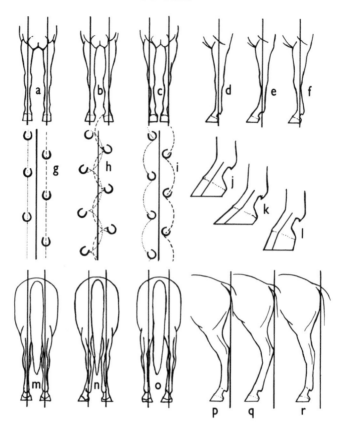

Leg conformation and travel

a. straight
b. toed-out
c. toed-in
d. straight
e. calf knee, camped out
f. buck knee
g. straight travel
h. winging in
i. paddling
j. aligned hoof-pastern axis

k. broken back axis
l. broken forward axis
m. straight
n. cow-hocked, toed-out
o. bowlegged, toed-in
p. correct
q. sickle hocked
r. post legged From *From the Center of the Ring* by Cherry Hill, Garden Way Publishing

the humerus, generally the higher the action; the more toward horizontal, the lower the action.

To evaluate the medial-lateral slope of the humerus from the front, find the left point of shoulder and (a spot in front of) the left point of elbow. Do the same on the right side. Connect the four points. If the resulting box is square, the humerus lies in an ideal position for straight lower limbs and straight travel. If the bottom of the box is wider, the horse may toe in and travel with loose elbows and paddle. If the bottom of the box is narrower, the horse will likely toe out, have tight elbows and wing in.

The way the shoulder blade and arm (humerus) are conformed and attach to the chest dictate, to a large degree, the alignment of the lower limbs. Whether the toes point in or out is often a result of upper limb structures. That is why it is dangerous in many cases to attempt to alter a limb's structure and alignment through radical hoof adjustments. When assessing the lower limbs, be sure the horse is standing square.

The knees should be large and clean, not small and puffy. The bone column should be functionally straight and sound, not buck-kneed or calf-kneed.

Normal front pastern angles range from 53 to 58 degrees. Exceptionally long, sloping pasterns can result in tendon strain, bowed tendons and damaged proximal sesamoids. Short, upright pasterns deliver greater concussive stresses to fetlock and pastern joints, which may result in osselets, ringbone and possibly navicular syndrome. Fetlock joints should be large enough to allow free movement, but they should be devoid of any puffiness. The hoof should be appropriate for the size of the horse, well shaped and symmetric, with high-quality hoof horn, adequate height and width of heel, a concave sole and adequate size hoof.

Hind limbs The bone structure and muscling of the hind limb should be appropriate for the intended use. Endurance horses are characterized by longer, flatter muscles; stock horses, by shorter, thicker muscles; all-around horses, by moderate muscles.

Limbs when viewed from the side should exhibit a composite of moderate angles, so that shock absorption will be efficient (see figure on page 100). A line from the point of buttock to the ground should touch the hock and end slightly behind the bulbs of the heels. A hind limb in front of this line is often sickle hocked; a hind limb behind this line is often postlegged or camped out.

The hindquarter should be symmetric and well connected to the barrel and the lower limb. The gluteals should tie well forward into the back. The hamstrings should tie down low into the Achilles tendon of the hock.

The relationship of the length of the bones, the angles of the joints and the overall height of the hind limb will dictate the type of action and the amount of power produced. The length and slope to the pelvis (croup) is measured from the point of hip to the point of buttock. A flat, level croup is associated with hind limb action that occurs *be-*

hind the hindquarters rather than underneath it. A goose rump is a very steep croup that places the hind limbs so far under the horse's belly that structural problems may occur due to the overangulation.

A short femur is associated with the short, rapid stride characteristic of a sprinter. A long femur results in a stride with more reach. High hocks are associated with snappy hock action and a difficulty getting the hocks under the body. Low hocks tend to have a smoother hock action, and the horse usually has an easier time getting the hocks under the body. The gaskin length (stifle to hock) should be shorter than the femur length (buttock to stifle). A gaskin longer than the femur tends to be associated with cow hocks and sickle hocks.

Hind limbs with open angles (a "straighter" hind limb when viewed from the side) have a shorter overall limb length and produce efficient movement suitable for hunters or race horses. Hind limbs with more closed joints (more angulation to the hind limb) have a longer overall limb length and produce a more vertical, folding action necessary for the collection characteristic of a high-level dressage horse. If the overall limb length is too long, however, it can be associated with either camped-out or sickle-hocked conformation. No matter what the hind limb conformation is at rest, however, it is the way it connects to the loin and operates in motion that is most important.

From the rear, both hind limbs should appear symmetric, to be of the same length and to bear equal weight. A left-to-right symmetry should be evident between the peaks of the croup, the points of the hip, the points of the buttock and the midline position of the tail. The widest point of the hindquarters should be the width between the stifles. A line dropped from the point of the buttock to the ground will essentially bisect the limb, but hind limbs are not designed to point absolutely straight forward. It is necessary and normal for the stifles to point slightly outward in order to clear the horse's belly. This causes the points of the hocks to face slightly inward and the toes to point outward to the same degree. The rounder the belly and/or the shorter the loin and coupling, the more the stifles must point out so the more the points of the hocks will appear to point inward. The more slab-sided and/or longer coupled a horse, the more straight ahead the stifles and hocks can point. When the cannon bone faces outward, the horse is often cow hocked; when cannons face inward, bowlegged.

Soundness problems can occur when the hocks point absolutely straight ahead and the hooves toe out; *then* there is stress on the hock and fetlock joints. The hind feet should be as far apart on the ground as the limbs are at their origin in the hip. Normal pastern angles for the hind range from 55 to 60 degrees.

SUPPORTING LIMB LAMENESS:

Head Movement at the Trot

Lame Limb	Head Down When These Limbs Land	Head Up When These Limbs Land
Right front	Left front/right hind	Right front/left hind
Left front	Right front/left hind	Left front/right hind
Right hind	Left front/right hind	Right front/left hind
Left hind	Right front/left hind	Left front/right hind

Although not absolute, the above is true in many cases. Note the potential confusion between right front and right hind supporting lamenesses and left front and left hind supporting lamenesses when using head movement at the trot as the sole indicator.

OTHER FACTORS THAT AFFECT MOVEMENT

Pain

Even if a horse shows conformational traits that theoretically are associated with straight travel, if he experiences a degree of pain in any portion of his body, he may break the conformation rules as he attempts to use his body in a manner that creates the least stress and pain. An injury or soreness in a limb or an associated structure can cause a horse to protect one portion of the limb when landing, subsequently altering the arc of the foot's flight. For example, if a horse is sore in the navicular region of his front feet, instead of landing heel first and rolling forward, he may land toe first, which will shorten his stride.

When a horse is off in a part of his body other than his hooves or limbs, his balance during movement may be negatively altered as he compensates for his pain or soreness. Back soreness can mimic a lower limb lameness and alter foot flight. A variety of other factors can cause the horse to carry his body in a stiff or crooked fashion: muscle cramping, a respiratory illness, a bad tooth, an ear infection, poor-fitting tack. Sometimes the stiffness or pain is low level but enough to prevent the horse from tracking straight.

Imbalance

Impure movement often occurs simply because the horse is trying to keep his balance. He is attempting to keep his limbs under his center of mass. Basically, there are three forces at work when a horse moves: the vertical force of the weight of the horse and rider; the horizontal force of the horse moving forward, and the swinging or side-to-side motion of the horse at various gaits. Exactly where under his body a horse places his limbs is determined in large part by the interaction of these three forces and the direction of their composite. A barefoot horse moving free in a pasture rarely interferes. It is when he carries a rider and is asked to perform in collected and extended frames and at both faster and slower speeds that interfering occurs.

A rider can make a horse move well or poorly. Rider proficiency will determine how the horse distributes his weight (from front to rear and from side to side), how the horse changes the speed of the stride or the length of a stride within a gait, how the horse adapts the stride when turning, stopping, and performing such maneuvers as lead changes. Inadequate riding skills exaggerate the deficiencies in a horse's conformation and way of going. Since no horse is perfect, or moves perfectly at all times, it takes a knowledgeable and competent rider to compensate for a horse's shortcomings. A rider's balance and condition as well as talent, coordination and skill at choosing and applying the aids greatly affect a horse's coordination. A horse must be warmed up in a progressive manner before asking him for more difficult work.

Inexperienced riders will often ask a cold or poorly conditioned horse to do three things at once, like come to a hard stop from a thundering gallop, make a sharp turn and lope off in the opposite direction, without properly preparing the horse or helping him perform in a balanced fashion. When a horse is asked to do something he is not physically ready to do such as a flying lead change, a deep stop, a fast burst out of the roping box, any kind of lateral work, a tight landing after a jump or a sharp turn, he can easily become imbalanced.

An unskilled rider can easily throw off a horse's balance formula. Inexperienced riders often commit one or more of these imbalance errors: sit off to one side of the saddle, often with a collapsed rib cage; ride with one stirrup longer; ride with a twisted pelvis; lean one shoulder lower than the other; hold one shoulder farther back than the other, or sit with a tilted head. All of these postures can affect the horse's composite center of mass and can cause the horse to make adjustments in order to stay balanced. Riders that let their horses

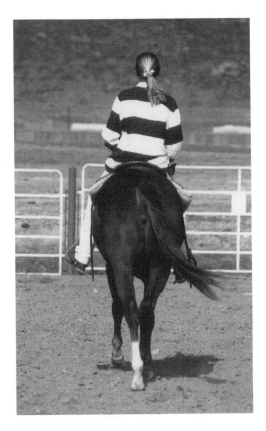

Rider imbalance

ramble in long, unbalanced frames, heavy on the forehand, also seem to have more forging problems. Some horses are able to compensate for an imbalanced rider without forging or interfering, others are not.

Some horses just have an imbalanced way of going. Certain horses are uncoordinated, inattentive and sloppy while others move precisely, gracefully and balanced. Training, conditioning and conscientious shoeing can improve a poor mover's tendencies, but some horses, no matter how talented the rider and farrier, will consistently move in an unbalanced fashion.

Shoeing

Recent but improper shoeing can be responsible for poor movement. If a farrier's shoeing style is "long-toe, low-heel," he sets the horse up to move poorly. A more common cause of movement impurities, however, is a horse being overdue for a reset. Even if the horse was shod by a world-class farrier eight weeks ago, his hooves have likely grown so out of balance that he could easily exhibit gait abnormalities. Sometimes just going a week past the horse's needs can adversely alter the gait synchronization (Chapters 4, 5, 9 and 11).

Footing

The surface the horse is worked on will directly affect his movement. Traction on dirt occurs when the horse's weight descends through the bone columns of the limbs, causing the hooves to drop ½ inch or more into the ground at the same time the soil is cupped upward toward the sole. This happens whether the horse is barefoot or shod. Shoes basically extend the hoof wall, creating a deeper cup to the bottom of the hoof and therefore increasing traction potential in dirt or soft footing.

Ideal arena footing is light and does not stay compressed, so most of it falls out of the hoof readily with every stride. During the work of a very active horse, the dirt literally flies out of the shoes, but a placid horse may not move its limbs energetically enough to release some

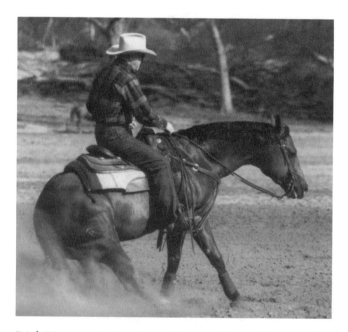

Dick Pieper training Texas Kicker, 1991 AQHA World Reining Champion Junior Reining horse, on his home track. Photo: Brenda Pieper

dirt with each stride. In dry arenas, the moderate amount of dirt in the shoe comes in contact with the dirt of the arena and results in good traction. However, if conditions are damp to wet, and the footing is heavy, the hooves may pack and mound, thereby decreasing stability and traction. Packed dirt left in for prolonged periods of time creates constant pressure on the sole and can cause sole and frog bruises. So for work in soft, wet and/or deep footing, it is important that shoes are self-cleaning; they should allow mud, manure or snow to pop out or move out at the base of the frog. This will ensure that the horse has an open sole and maximum traction potential for each stride. This self-cleaning is facilitated by concaving the inner edge of the ground surface of the shoe (see figure on page 32). Some performance events have specialized footing requirements and it is important that a horse is trained at home on the most ideal footing possible.

Heavy footing (sand, mud, snow, long grass) generally delays front foot breakover. If a horse must be worked on footing he is unaccustomed to, protective boots may be helpful. Bell boots and scalping boots may prevent injury to the heels and coronary bands. Overreach boots will provide protection to the tendons. "Splint boots" will help protect the inner surface of the leg when interference is a problem. (See Resource Guide in the Appendix.)

Traction

In some instances, a horse requires greater traction than would be provided by a standard shoe: an extreme example is tall studs for jumping. Generally, the wider the web of the shoe, the less traction the shoe will provide. The most extreme example of this is the reining horse's sliding plate, which can be over 1 inch wide and allows the horse to "float" over the ground surface.

Optimum traction can increase horse and rider safety, increase a horse's feeling of security so he will stride normally, and can help a horse maintain his balance in unstable footing such as mud, ice, snow or rock (Chapter 10).

Condition, Level of Fitness

A horse's overall level of fitness as well as his present energy level will affect his movement. In general, a horse has fifteen minutes of peak performance whether in a daily work session or at a competition. He is either approaching that peak period or coming away from it. A rider must know how to properly warm up a horse to establish the most natural and efficient way of going for that horse; then he must assist, not hinder, the horse in working in a balanced frame during the peak period; and finally a rider must know how to gradually let the horse come down from his peak. A horse predisposed to forge or overreach may likely do so if he is allowed to dawdle around on the forehand during the warm-up, if the bridle reins are pulled up suddenly and the horse is put to work when he is "cold," if contact is "thrown away" all at once or engagement is allowed to slip away during work, or if the horse is allowed to fall on his forehand immediately following the completion of his peak performance.

If a rider asks too much in relation to a horse's current physical capabilities or fitness level, many horses will adapt, attempting to comply. If overworked, many horses will continue moving forward but will modify stride to minimize fatigue and discomfort to flexor muscles and tendons. When a tired horse adjusts the timing of the various phases of its stride, it can result in gait defects. If the hindquarters have not been properly conditioned and strengthened, a horse will rely heavily on the forehand for both propulsion and support. This makes it even harder for the already heavily weighted forehand to get out of the way of the incoming hind feet.

Poor condition or fatigue will often cause a horse to fling his limbs aimlessly—he does not have the muscle strength or energy necessary to project his limbs in a controlled fashion. In some cases, when a lazy horse moves slowly at a trot, he may move sloppily and carelessly, and this may cause him to occasionally interfere. Requiring such a horse to move out with more energy may smooth out gait defects. This situation can be interpreted as an exception to the general rule that an increase in speed usually brings an increase in the potential to interfere. The amount of weight a horse is carrying can also exaggerate its lateral limb movements. An overweight horse or heavy rider may cause more side-to-side sway, which will alter the net forward movement.

Age and Stage of Development

Young horses that do not have fully developed muscles may lack the width of chest, stifle or hip necessary for straightforward, efficient movement. For example, the relationship between the inside and outside muscles can affect how the limb swings. A horse with heavy outside gaskin muscling and, in comparison, light inside gaskin muscling, especially if his hind limbs toe out, will tend to have trouble keeping his limbs under his body during a stop, which can be a major problem for a stock horse. There simply isn't enough inside gaskin muscle power to counteract the outward rotation of the limb during the stop.

Training

One of the main causes of poor movement and intermittent gait defects is asking a horse to perform something beyond his level of training. One of the first goals of training is to teach a horse to track straight. Until a horse learns to strongly and decisively step up underneath himself, his travel is often wobbly and inconsistent. Working on circles and lateral maneuvers before a horse is balanced and supple can cause him to make missteps and interfere. Asking a horse to perform advanced movements like the passage, canter pirouette or turnaround before the horse is physically developed and trained can increase the possibility of interference and/or injury. These movements are characterized by either higher action, greater speed or a greater degree of joint flexion, all of which tend to increase rotational forces of the limb and the possibility of interference. Gait defects tend to surface with an increase in speed within a gait as well as the extension of a stride within a gait.

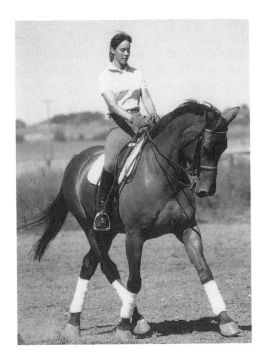

Proper training prevents missteps during advanced lateral work. Margot Dippert on Zoro

Tack

A poor-fitting saddle is one of the main causes of back pain and subsequently poor movement. If a tree is too narrow, it will perch on the horse's back and cause pinching of the nerves and muscular pain. If the tree is too wide, it places the weight of the saddle and rider directly on the vertebrae. If the balance of the saddle causes the rider's weight to be borne by a small area at the withers, the withers may become injured and result in poor forelimb movement. If the saddle is imbalanced to the rear, and especially if the saddle is very long, the loin bears most of the weight, and this can lead to back and hind limb problems.

Other Factors

A host of other factors can cause a horse to move in an irregular fashion. Some mares move with stiffness and tension during a portion of their estrous cycle. Horses with dental problems often carry their head and neck in an unnatural position, which affects their overall movement. A sour, balky or otherwise ill-tempered animal moves with characteristic resistance.

Become involved in analyzing your horse's problem. Begin with an objective assessment of his conformation. Then watch and listen as the horse is led and ridden on a smooth, level surface in a straight line at a walk and trot. View the horse from the front, rear and side. Use a camera with high-speed shutter to film your horse's movement. Carefully consider all factors that can affect movement. If poor or irregular shoeing is the obvious factor at fault, remedy it. Do the same with any deficiencies in the horse's training or management before looking to corrective or therapeutic shoeing treatment.

C H A P T E R 9

Dealing with Gait Defects

The straight foot flight pattern that is used as a basis when talking about deviations has often been termed ideal. The fact is, such a foot flight is ideal only for a horse with ideal body and limb conformation. Horses with imperfections in their structural components, which includes virtually all horses, will each have their own "ideal" foot flight patterns that compensate for their individual imperfections. While a particular horse's pattern may not be "text-book pretty," it may be the most functional and efficient for that horse. Instead of thinking of the straight foot flight as "ideal," think of it as "straight," so that rather than representing a goal, the term indicates a baseline for comparison.

Straight front limb movement starts with a straight bone column and a series of hinge joints all symmetrically conformed and working in a true forward-backward plane. Add to this a balanced hoof and the result should be a straight foot flight (see figure on page 100). Since hind limbs nearly always turn out to some degree (Chapter 8), hind limbs tend to wing in slightly.

GAIT DEFECTS

Gait defects are abnormalities in movement that consistently occur during regular work. Lateral gait defects (inward or outward swing of a limb) can affect a pair of limbs or a single limb. Conformational components that should be evaluated include (in the front limb, for example) shoulder to rib cage attachment; width of chest; width of knees, fetlock and hoof; and straightness of forearm, cannon, pastern and hoof.

The underdevelopment (hypoplasia) of one portion of a joint surface (usually of the knee or fetlock joint) can also cause a limb to exhibit a lateral gait defect. Normally the fetlock and knee joints work in a hingelike fashion, backward and forward in a straight line, parallel with the horse's midline. A hypoplastic joint appears to hinge in a swivel-like motion at an angle to the horse's midline. This arc causes the limb to deviate in flight.

Gait defects involving timing and length of stride are related to how close a horse's front and hind feet come together when the horse is moving. Factors to consider when evaluating these defects include the relationship between height at the wither and height at the hip;

DEFECTS IN TRAVEL

Paddling   The foot is thrown *outward* in flight, but the foot often lands *inside* the normal track. Often associated with wide and/or toed-in conformation. Unsightly but rarely causes interference.

Winging   The foot swings *inward* in flight but often lands *outside* the normal track. Often associated with narrow and/or toed-out conformation. Dangerous because it can result in interfering.

Plaiting   Also called rope-walking, the horse places one foot directly in front of the other; dangerous due to stumbling and tripping; can be associated with chest-narrow, base-narrow, toed-out conformation or chest-wide, base-narrow, toed-in conformation.

Interfering   Striking a limb with the opposite limb. Associated with toed-out, base-narrow conformation. Results in tripping, wounds.

Forging   Hitting the sole or the shoe of the forefoot with the toe of the hind foot on the same side. Associated with low withers and high hip (downhill conformation); sickle hocks with a short back and long limbs; a tired, young or unconditioned horse, one that needs reset or one who has long toes and low heels.

Overreaching   Hitting the heel of the forefoot (or other portions of the limb or hoof) with the hind foot on the same side before the forefoot has left the ground. Also called grabbing. Often results in wounds and lost shoes. Associated with the same factors listed in forging.

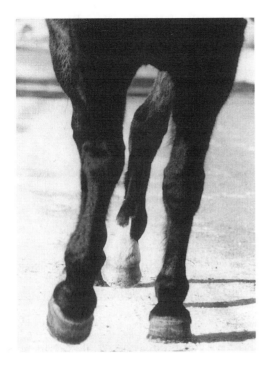

Paddling

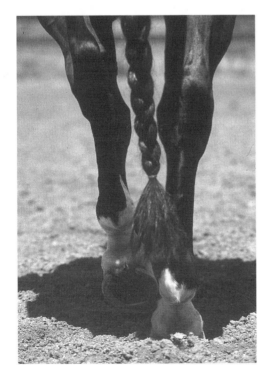

Winging

the amount of muscling and the width of the chest and hips; the length, proportion and shape of topline components; the relationship between the length of the topline to the length of the underline; the relationship between the length of underline to the length of his limbs. Horses with downhill conformation or short backs and long limbs, and those with short front limbs and long hind limbs, are the most likely to have contact between front and hind limbs.

Forging

Forging is a gait defect most commonly detected when a horse is trotting. Forging customarily refers to contact made between a hind toe (hoof or shoe) and a front sole or the toe of a front shoe on the same side. Frequently the contact is made when the hind foot is gliding in for a landing and the front foot is between breakover and the swing phase (Chapter 7). If the front foot is delayed in its break-

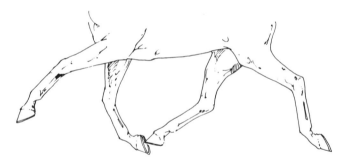

Forging at the trot

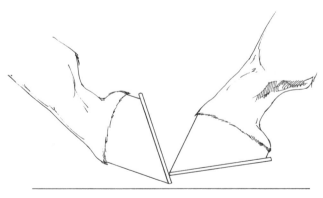

Close up of forging at the trot

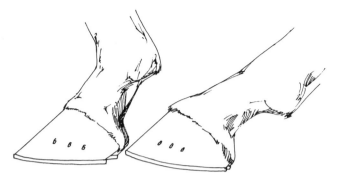

The moment a shoe might be "grabbed" when the front foot is greatly delayed in breakover.

over, the hind foot may arrive before the front foot has a chance to get out of the way. As the fetlock of the front foot begins to hinge, the hoof may swing back and slap the toe of the incoming hind hoof. This creates the characteristic click-click when a shod horse forges at the trot and a dull thwack-thwack if he is barefoot. A horse can receive sole bruises from a single hard blow or repeated low-intensity contact.

Overreaching usually indicates that a front shoe has been "grabbed" or pulled off by a hind or that the hind has injured some part of the front limb, such as the heel, bulb, coronary band or even the fetlock or flexor tendons. A horse that forges or overreaches may be more prone to stumble or fall, especially at the moment when the shoe is stepped on or pulled off. If the conditions that cause a horse to forge are ignored or inadvertently perpetuated, the stride imbalances may progress to over-reaching.

Forging and over-reaching are indications that the horse's movement is out of balance (Chapters 5 and 7). Balance can refer to the relationship between the front and rear of the horse's entire body as well as to the relationship between each hoof and pastern (DP balance). Balance also involves the relationship between the left and right sides of the horse's body. Most horses have an inherent left-right (LR) imbalance, which can cause stiff or crooked movement. Medial-lateral (ML) imbalances of hooves and limbs occur most frequently in the knees, hocks, fetlocks and hoofs and are implicated as causes of gait defects such as winging in and paddling (covered later in this chapter). Although LR and ML imbalances can complicate the forging or overreaching horse's problems, these gait defects are mainly due to DP imbalances.

Causes of Forging A horse's balance during movement is influenced by many factors (Chapter 8) that can affect breakover. The *theoretical* discussion of breakover deals with the function of one limb at a time. However, to correct forging, the timing and direction of breakover of *all* of the hooves must be coordinated so the limbs work in harmony and avoid collision.

Forging Solutions Breakover is the phase of the stride between stance and swing when the hoof is preparing to leave the ground. The balanced hoof will break over near the center of the toe. The location of breakover is different for front and hind hooves. Since the coffin bone and hoof of a front foot are round with sloping hoof walls and wide areas of support on each side of the hoof, breakover usually occurs at the center of the toe. That's why front shoes usually show the most wear at the toe.

Hind hooves are pointed and triangular in shape, with straighter walls and less lateral support. They are the horse's means to push, pivot and change direction, so perform a wide variety of medial-lateral movements. Most horses normally toe out to some degree in the hind. Therefore, hind hooves (and shoes) often do not break over at the center of the toe, but slightly to the inside. Instead of showing wear at the point of breakover, however, hind shoes usually show a more even wear from sliding and swiveling on the ground.

In most cases, the point of breakover should not be *forced* to occur at a point that is unnatural for the individual horse. However, a hoof can be *encouraged* to break over in a position that will contribute to balanced movement. If a horse's hooves are balanced, he is most likely breaking over at his ideal spot.

Providing that a horse's hoof is aligned with the pastern, some correlations can be drawn between angles and breakover. Longer or lower pasterns (53 degrees or lower) result in the hoof being on the ground for a longer period of time than those with shorter or more upright (59 degrees or higher) pasterns.

The length and position of the hoof's base of support in relation to the cannon and fetlock will determine how much time and effort it will take to break over. A hoof (or shoe) is in the proper position to support a horse's weight if the heels contact the ground approximately beneath the midpoint of the cannon bone when the horse is standing on all four limbs and the cannon is vertical. Hooves that are small or have underrun heels (and are not shod to counteract this) will sink more at the heels during loading and therefore will experience more stress, require more effort to lift and have a delayed breakover. Egg bar or extended heel shoes minimize the backward sinking of the hoof at the heel, therefore the hoof is in position to spring up more quickly and easily.

Dishes or extra length of toe, if not removed, will increase the length of the lever arm, increase tendon stress and delay breakover. If a dish is not rasped to result in a straight hoof wall from the coronary band to the ground, the shoe will probably be applied ahead of the optimum point of breakover.

Assuming management and training factors have been evaluated and modified if required, shoeing may be able to help eliminate the problem of persistent forging or over-reaching. Most corrective shoeing is based on restoring a horse's normal hoof configuration and balance.

There are no absolutes when it comes to corrective shoeing for forging or overreaching. While most experts agree how to modify the front feet of a horse that forges or overreaches, the opinions are varied for treatment of the hinds. Often just balancing the front hooves and easing their breakover will eliminate forging. This balancing is usually accomplished by shortening the toe and/or raising the hoof angle to align the hoof/pastern axis. Breakover can be eased with a modified toe shoe (Chapter 6).

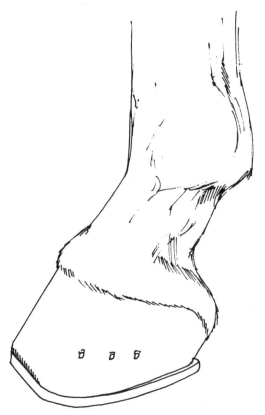

Squared-toe shoe

The DP balance of the rear hooves should be evaluated and adjusted, if necessary. In the case of a horse that is relatively equal in
width of chest and hindquarters, putting a modified toe shoe, such as
a squared-toe shoe, on the hinds as well as the fronts might eliminate
forging. Why would this work, since the breakover of both the fronts
and hinds has been made easier (quicker)? In the case of a horse with
a very pointed hind hoof, sometimes squaring the front hooves and
leaving the hinds pointed would result in a break in the synchronization of the movement of the diagonal pairs of limbs. Squaring the
hind toes may smooth out and equalize the movement. And the
square toe on the hind replaces the normally pointed hind toe; a
pointed toe would tend to hit and perhaps grab a front shoe more
easily than a squared toe would. Using half-round or rocker toe shoes
on the hinds, or the fronts and hinds, may also be helpful.

To prevent pulled shoes due to overreaching, many farriers remove the sharp outer edges of the shoes. Chamfering the outer edge
of the hoof surface of the shoe is called boxing, and rounding the
outer edge of the ground surface of the shoe is called safeing (see
figure on page 32). Two rounded surfaces (in contrast to two square-
edged surfaces) are less likely to grab onto each other and result in a
lost shoe. (Half-round and some rim shoes already have a rounded
ground surface.)

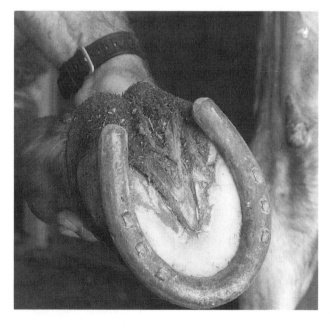

Half-round shoe

Trailers have long been touted as an aid to encourage a hoof to stop sooner on landing if the hoof is meeting the ground heel first or flat. However, a smooth trailer increases the surface area of the shoe and actually provides less traction. A calk or sticker on the trailer *would* contact the ground sooner and create additional drag, but the trailer just provides a place for the calk to be placed. It is the calk that is doing the stopping, not the trailer. This is where the confusion may have originated.

Even if trailers on the hinds *did* encourage a slightly quicker stop to the hoof's motion as it lands, would it prevent forging or over-reaching? According to some slow-motion videos and photos, the answer is no. The moment when contact between the toe of the hind and the front shoe would occur is when the hind is gliding in for a landing (usually flat or toe first) before the hind shoe (and its smooth trailers) touches the ground. Trailers do offer a greater measure of support for the flexor tendons than normal shoes. However, exaggerated trailers can be dangerous to people and other horses in the event of a kick and fatal for horses turned out with halters on. Egg bar shoes are a safer alternative for providing extension for support.

Interfering

A lateral gait defect is one that involves a regularly occurring, abnormal sideways swing of a limb. Some lateral gait defects result in actual physical contact with an opposite limb. Others do not. Paddling or dishing, often seen with bow-legged, toed-in or wide-chested and base-narrow horses, is a swinging out of the limb from the midline, so contact rarely results.

In contrast, interfering is frequently associated with narrow and/or toed-out horses. Such chest conformation places the limbs closer together, and the toed-out hoof predisposes the horse to winging or brushing, that is, swinging the limb toward the midline during flight. As one limb swings inward, it passes the opposite limb, which is in a weight-bearing position. It is at this moment when contact might occur. The higher up the limb the turned-out deviation is located, the greater the torque imparted to the limb and the worse the winging will likely be.

Interfering rarely occurs at the walk. It appears most commonly at the trot, canter and back. The speed and energy level with which a horse moves its limbs will have an effect on its tendency to interfere. One horse may interfere at the jog but not at the extended trot; another horse may move with adequate clearance at the jog but not at an energetic trot. Similarly, one horse performing a quiet rein-back might move his limbs carefully, but when asked to speed up the back, his limbs might swing from side to side and collide. Another horse may work his limbs with pistonlike precision while backing quickly and straight, but might exhibit a clumsy, uncoordinated foot flight if asked to slow down.

Interference can occur from the knee to the hoof of the front limbs and usually from the fetlock to the hoof of the hind limbs. If a horse does not wear protective boots, the first signs of interference may be pain, heat or swelling in the area of contact. The problem may escalate to include missing hair, bruises, cuts, lesions, chronic sores and perhaps underlying bone damage.

Protective boots should be used, examined and cleaned after each workout and points of contact noted. However, just because contact was made with a boot or leg wrap does not mean that contact would have been made without the protective gear, because the thickness of the boot may be the safe tolerance in which the unbooted horse would work. Rather than take a chance of injury, however, it is best to use protective boots on all young horses and older horses whose conformation or performance requirements point to the possibility of interference. (See Resource Guide in the Appendix.)

Sometimes a horse will show reluctance to perform certain maneuvers that have caused him to hit himself in the past. He may try to avoid circular or lateral work by stiffening the back, and working

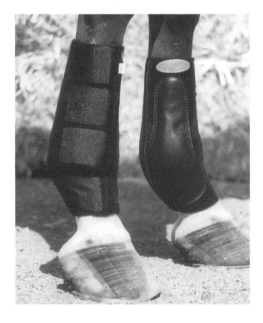

Protective boots. Photo: Pro Equine

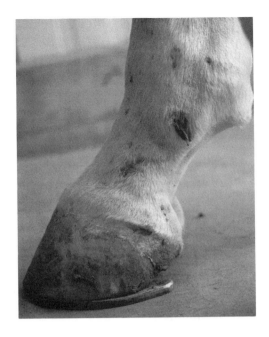

Interference marks on hind limbs

with short hopping strides with the hind limbs. With a reining horse, interference problems in the front limbs may make him reluctant to add speed to his turnaround.

Interference Adjustments Why a horse interferes can be due to a variety of factors (Chapter 8). In some cases, finding a solution requires the trainer, farrier and perhaps a veterinarian to work together during a period of trial and error.

First, a knowledgeable farrier should examine the horse's shoes for signs of imbalance. Shoe wear, which is related to the hoof landing, loading and taking off, is valuable information for assessing a foot flight problem. The torque, or twisting force, that the deviating foot experiences and expresses in flight, is a direct result of the impact of loading and the way the horse's weight is released during breakover. If a hoof lands unbalanced, it usually sends the energy upward and forward in an unbalanced fashion, and the flight of the limb and/or hoof will show a resulting deviation. In general, the goal is a balanced hoof and even weight bearing, which will usually result in even shoe wear.

If the hoof is obviously unbalanced, then alterations in trimming and shoeing should come first. Otherwise, conscientious corrections to all riding, conditioning and training deficiencies should be made *before* turning to farriery for additional solutions to the interference problems. Shoeing alterations should be approached conservatively and monitored closely. One of the most serious misconceptions surrounding corrective farriery is the notion that crooked limbs should be made to point forward. While there can be merit to this in the developing young horse, forcing a foot to conform to an "ideal" on a horse over one year of age often results in serious stress to joint alignment and function. Forcing a horse's feet to point forward to deceive a halter judge into thinking that a horse has good genes is unethical and inhumane.

With a toed-out condition, it is not uncommon for the bones from the fetlock to the coffin bone to be aligned in a desirable, straight column with even, symmetric joint spaces but with the entire column rotated outward instead of straight forward. If alteration (commonly a lowering of the outside) forces the hoof to point forward, then joint spaces on the inside of the joints become tighter (closer), while the joint spaces on the outside of the joints become looser (farther apart). Now there *is* a problem.

When farrier corrections are warranted, they can affect the breakover, flight, landing and/or weight bearing of the hoof. Some interference problems will require experimentation over a period of several shoeings before a pattern begins to emerge and the solution materializes. Unfortunately, a small number of horses will continue to interfere in spite of the best management, riding, training and farrier care.

Breakover A squared or rocker toe shoe can be located to encourage the breakover to occur off center if desired. Often it is necessary to experiment during several shoeing periods to find the optimum breakover that will help an interfering horse. It is usually better to *encourage* breakover at a desired point than to *prevent* breakover at

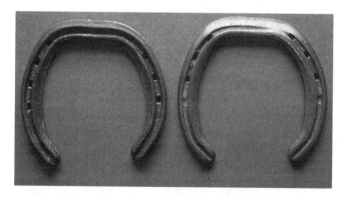

From left: New offset squared-toe shoe and worn offset squared-toe shoe

an undesirable point. However, in some cases, toe extensions are appropriate. A toe extension is a metal piece forged or welded to a particular portion of the shoe to inhibit breakover at that point. To prevent interference, toe extensions are used on the inside of a base-narrow, toed-out horse to help the horse break over centrally. The extension is added from the center of the toe of the shoe to approximately the second nail hole.

Half-round shoes, polo shoes and rim shoes allow breakover in any direction, so are inappropriate to use when trying to redirect the breakover, but they will allow a horse to more easily find this natural breakover point.

Foot Flight In order to affect the natural flight of a hoof as little as possible, it is best to use the lightest shoe that will still provide adequate support for the hoof. If the foot flight pattern of the front feet needs to be widened, lowering the outside wall and possibly adding a calk on the inside may work. If the foot flight pattern of the hind feet of a cow-hocked horse needs to be widened, lowering the outside wall and adding a trailer on the outside and a calk on the inside may work. If the foot flight pattern of the hind feet of a base-narrow or bowlegged horse needs to be widened, lowering the inside wall and adding a calk on a trailer on the outside may work. Bear in mind, however, that by lowering one side of a hoof that is in balance to affect foot flight or by using calks on only one branch of a shoe, the limb's support structures experience uneven stress and may experience problems worse than interfering.

Undesirable torque in flight is usually due to an unbalanced foot or misaligned limb. Joint rotation, such as seen in the bowlegged or knock-kneed horse, increases as speed or extension within a gait increases. Sometimes the foot flight pattern can be improved by applying the shoes so they are in line with the horse's body regardless how the hoofs point.

Some Standardbred farriers use side-weighted shoes to control knee torque and alter foot flight. Weight affects front and hind limbs differently. Added weight on a front foot tends to move the limb away from the weighted side. Added weight on a hind foot tends to pull the limb toward the weighted side. However, these principles are more appropriate for high-speed or high-action horses than for horses moving at normal gaits.

Landing Encouraging a hoof to land in a balanced fashion begins with trimming the hoof level and shoeing it to land flat or slightly heel first. If alterations to landing are desired, they are usually accomplished by altering the balance of the hoof. Extending or shortening one heel of the shoe so that both heels land simultaneously may improve the movement of some horses. Trailers and/or calks on one heel of a shoe are sometimes used to turn the hoof upon landing, but as previously mentioned calks, especially when used singly, are considered by many to be dangerous because of the uneven stresses they put on the structures of the limb.

Weight Bearing Ideally during the loading phase of the stride, the horse's weight is borne over the center of the hoof. If a horse shows a dynamic imbalance in weight bearing, an attempt to move the hoof under the center of the limb can be made by raising up or lowering the pertinent side of the hoof. Lowering the lateral (outer) wall will move the hoof toward the midline, while lowering the medial (inner) wall will move the hoof away from the midline. If the hoof is balanced but offset on the leg, a farrier will often approach the situation by placing the shoe on the hoof so that the *shoe* is under the center of the limb. In this case, the shoe would fit close on one side of the hoof and extend beyond the hoof on the other side.

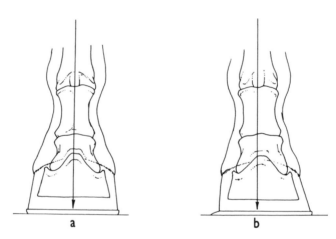

Base of support centered under limb
a. Centered hoof
b. Offset hoof

Paddling

Wide-chested and/or toed-in conformation is associated with paddling, where the foot is thrown outward in flight but often lands inside the normal track. Often, balancing the hooves and encouraging breakover to occur where the hoof "wants" to break over will diminish paddling. If paddling continues once the hooves are balanced, yet the horse is sound and does not interfere, paddling should be considered normal movement for that horse. It would be foolish to put uneven stress on a limb by means of trimming, calks or wedges to "fix" something that is not a problem.

Shoeing for Your Event

No matter what style of riding you prefer or what event you enjoy participating in, your horse should be shod following the guidelines outlined under Preventive Shoeing in Chapter 5. Your horse's soundness and comfort must be the first priorities, and these can only be achieved by trimming and shoeing the hoof in balance and alignment and as naturally as possible.

For the most part, the quality of a horse's performance is determined by his inherent talent and heart and the correctness of his training and riding. Shoeing can allow the horse to perform to his best, but shoeing should not be thought of as a means to *make* a horse perform in a certain way. The top trainers and farriers of horses in many disciplines often voice a version of this thought: The training of a horse does not start at the bottom of his foot, but conscientious shoeing will provide the horse with the opportunity to perform at his best in a balanced fashion.

Most breed and performance organizations have rules related to shoes, pads and hoof length. If you are planning to compete in a specific event, follow the current rules and discuss their application with your farrier.

DRESSAGE

Nowhere is shoeing for balance and support more important than with the dressage horse. Dressage is a means of systematically training a horse through progressive developmental stages. The rider's goals are a forward, free-moving horse that is supple and submissive,

LAMENESSES GENERALLY ASSOCIATED WITH SPECIFIC ACTIVITIES

Event	Movement	Lameness
Dressage	Sitting trot	Back
	Weight carried rearward	Hip
	Increased joint flexion	Early hock arthritis, bone
	Great impulsion	spavin
	Collection	Stifle inflammation (gonitis)
	Extension	Fetlock arthritis
Reining	Deep, sliding stops	Hamstring tear, short pastern
	Fast spins	bone fracture hind
	Rollbacks	Early hock arthritis, bone spavin
Cutting	Balancing and turning on hindquarters with power and torque	Front bruised soles, long and short pastern bone fractures Early hock arthritis, bone spavin Gonitis
Roping	Explosive bursts	Short pastern and coffin bone
	Hard stops and jerks	fractures, bone spavin
		Navicular syndrome
Racing (TB & QH)	Young horses	Bucked shins
	Top speed	Fatigue fractures
	Footing stresses	Bowed tendons
	Fatigue	Carpitis
		Carpal chip and slab fractures
		Suspensory ligament injuries
		Fetlock arthritis and chip fractures
		Sesamoid fractures
Barrel racing Pole bending	Speed with turning, torque and twist	Fetlock arthritis Coffin bone fractures Ligament sprain Navicular syndrome Ringbone
Show ring	Repetitive circular and arena work, often on hard footing	Navicular syndrome Sprain trauma to fetlock and long and short pastern bones

Event	Movement	Lameness
Jumping	Fetlock hyperextension	Navicular syndrome
Eventing	Landing after jump	Bowed tendon
	Cross country footing	Ligament sprain
	Too much/too little traction	
Endurance	Long miles	Bowed tendons
	Often hard or rocky footing	Coffin bone inflammation
	Fatigue	Hoof injuries
		Sole bruises
		Fatigue fractures
Inactivity	Lack of movement	Laminitis
	Poor blood flow	Contracted heels
	Overweight	
Confinement	Explosive exercising	Trauma injuries
then turnout	Sudden outbursts	

calm but keen and responsive to light contact without resistance or resentment. The elegance and harmony between horse and rider takes years to develop and perfect. Since it takes so long to train a dressage horse, it is especially important that no compromises to his long-term soundness be made to rush his progress or enhance his immediate performance. A great degree of control and precision are required to execute the movements in dressage so it is important that the dressage horse be confident in his footing and that he has an adequate base of support (Chapter 5).

Plain, wide web, or rim shoes usually provide the traction necessary for dressage (Chapters 4 and 6). Calks are rarely used because they interfere with the horse's natural movement and place unnecessary stress on the limbs. Full pads are also used with a great deal of discretion, since they reduce a horse's traction and negatively affect his confidence, especially on turns in a wet arena. Aluminum shoes are seldom used on dressage horses because steel shoes hold up better under the larger, heavier horses that are used in dressage. A young horse is often shod with a half-round or rim shoe to allow free movement in all directions. As his muscles develop and his hoof size increases, he can move into a wider-web shoe that offers more support.

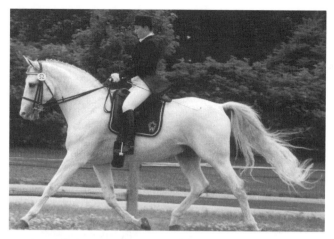

Extended trot. Chronos, ridden by Susan Wallen.
Photo: D. Kay Klein

As with other sports, if a dressage horse has mismatched feet, he is shod to balance his *movement,* not to balance the *appearance* of his hooves. That is, he is balanced dynamically, not statically.

Egg Bar Shoes Egg bar shoes are commonly used for dressage horses not only to provide support for weak hooves but as a preventive measure on sound hooves. The egg bar shoe should not be thought of as just a *therapeutic* shoe but as a *preventive* shoe as well (Chapter 6). In many cases, an egg bar is not a red flag signaling an unsoundness but a green flag indicating that the trainer and farrier recognize the importance of support for longevity. The egg bar shoe is being used with increasing frequency as a performance enhancer, soundness protector and lameness preventive.

The work of a dressage horse is characteristically energetic and comprised of greater-than-average vertical loading forces. Dressage horses at all levels are asked to move with a great deal of forward energy. The more active the forward motion, the greater the loading of the limbs on impact and therefore the greater the stress on flexor tendons. And as a horse moves up in the levels and begins the collected movements (the collected trot and canter, the pirouette and the piaffe and passage) the work results in even *more* vertical forces on the limbs. The joints exhibit a higher degree of flexion and the limbs move in a more upward/downward plane than the horizontal plane characteristic of lower-level movements.

As a horse progresses in his training, his center of balance shifts rearward. The horse is asked to carry more weight with his hindquarters and for longer periods of time. His muscles, joints, and support structures are conditioned gradually to accept this new work load. The additional support of egg bar shoes helps to compensate for the rearward weight shift. (Extended shoes are also helpful in this regard, but it is important that the heels are not so long that they result in interference when the horse crosses over in lateral movements.)

Although efforts have been made to standardize and improve footing at dressage competitions, there are still situations where the footing is deep, uneven or slippery. Egg bar shoes help minimize tendon strain exacerbated by poor footing.

The egg bar shoe's increased popularity is due to the greater demands put on today's dressage horses, the growing awareness of the potential support benefits of the shoe and the positive effect the shoe

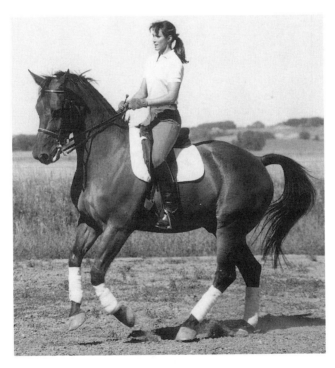

A moment in the pirouette. Zoro, ridden by Margot Dippert. From *Becoming an Effective Rider* by Cherry Hill, Garden Way Publishing

can have on the domesticated hoof of today's horse. Due to the time and money required to produce and develop a top-notch dressage horse, riders should be concerned with long-term soundness.

WESTERN PLEASURE

A Western Pleasure horse should look like he is enjoyable and comfortable to ride, and he should move soundly and correctly at all gaits. The gaits should be performed at a moderate speed so they are pure gaits: a four-beat walk, a two-beat trot and a three-beat lope. Western Pleasure movement should be efficient, characterized by a "flat knee" (very little knee flexion) and a "quiet hock" (very little hock flexion). The drive from the hindquarters comes from a strong but relaxed and supple back that hinges at the loin, resulting in the hind legs being able to work well under the body. The Western Pleasure horse should travel square, not with his hind legs offset to the travel of his front legs.

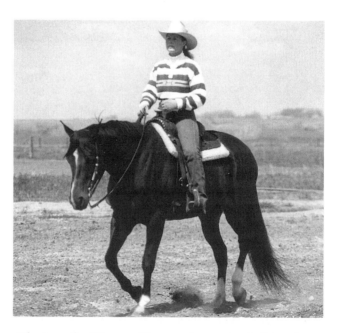

The jog of a Western Pleasure horse. Carla Wennberg, rider. From *Becoming an Effective Rider* by Cherry Hill, Garden Way Publishing

Good preventive shoeing (Chapter 5) is all that most talented western pleasure horses require. Aluminum shoes are used on some horses to help keep their stride smooth and low and to minimize knee and hock action.

SHOW HUNTER

A good hunter course has a flowing, smooth path with no sharp turns. There usually is at least one change of direction requiring a change of lead. The hunter must negotiate the course with a steady, moderate pace exhibiting adequate length of stride and good timing. To score well, the hunter must use his body in a rhythmic, smooth manner and negotiate each fence with style and confidence. Hunter movement on the flat is characterized by a long, low frame with a horizontal, gliding movement. There should be little knee and hock flexion as the limbs swing forward, resulting in the hooves appearing to "clip the daisies." To encourage this movement and to provide the security necessary for negotiating a course, the show hunter is shod following *preventive* principles and with these special considerations.

One guideline to keep in mind is that the heavier the shoe, generally the higher the action of the limbs. Therefore, to keep the swing phase of the hunter's stride low to the ground, the front hooves are shod with the lightest shoes that will still provide adequate support. Many horses perform well as hunters with plain steel shoes. The stride of some horses can be lowered by using aluminum or titanium shoes, particularly on the front (Chapters 6 and 8).

Some farriers provide a lighter shoe by modifying a factory-made wide-web steel shoe or a forged full-creased shoe made from ¼- or ⁵⁄₁₆ by ⅞-inch bar stock. The inside edge of the ground surface of the shoe is chamfered with a grinder, making the shoe concave in profile (see figure on page 32). This lightens a large steel shoe by as much as 4 ounces without significantly reducing its strength. The resulting cupped shape of the shoe also provides more traction than a flat, wide-web shoe, and such a shoe self-cleans more readily.

The hinds of hunters are frequently shod with a rim shoe to provide a gentle grip, traction that is appropriate for a normal hunter performance in the arena or in the field. If performance will likely be in wet footing and it is necessary to provide the horse with a greater degree of traction, the shoes can be drilled and tapped for screw-in studs. For more information on studs, see Shoeing the Jumper later in this chapter.

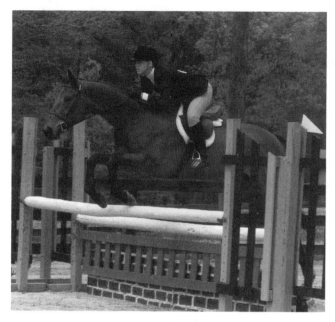

*Show hunter. Shadowfax, ridden by student Paige
Tomberlin, Sweet Briar College, Sweet Briar, Virginia.*
Photo: © Al Cook

Extended heels or trailers on the hind shoes will provide a wider
support base and may help the horse negotiate corners more confidently. (Some farriers use a trailer or extended heel only on the lateral branch of the shoe.)

The toes of the hind shoes are often squared to prevent injury to
the front heel bulbs in case of overreaching and to minimize the risk
of the hind toe stepping off a front shoe.

Many of the horses used as show ring hunters are Thoroughbreds,
and they often inherit challenging hooves. These hooves tend to be
wide across the quarters, have low heels, flat soles and thin walls. It
is important that the toe length be controlled on this type of hoof and
that strong, healthy heels are encouraged so the hoof/pastern angle
can be aligned and maintained. Although toe lengths vary among
horses, 3¼ to 3½ inches is a common length for a normal-sized
hunter. It is not uncommon for hunters to perform well wearing egg
bar or full support shoes on the fronts, hinds or all four hooves if
necessary. Steel bar shoes may cause an undesirable increase in some
horse's action, in which case aluminum bar shoes may be better.

If a hunter requires pads due to flat or thin soles, it might be best to use them with aluminum or titanium shoes. These light shoes will offset the extra weight of the pad and packing. The pad will also prevent the aluminum from reacting with the hoof wall. "Pour in" pads, which are applied to the sole after the hoof is shod, are available. These pads can protect the sole without increasing hoof length. Clips are very useful in maintaining the Thoroughbred-type foot and are essential if using pads (Chapter 6).

ENGLISH PLEASURE

The term English Pleasure encompasses a wide variety of performance classes. Here English Pleasure will refer to horses shod naturally and exhibited on the flat at a walk, trot and canter under Saddle Seat tack and attire.

English Pleasure horses customarily enter the ring at a normal trot performed at medium speed and with moderate collection. The walk must be a pure, four-beat gait that is flat footed and exhibits good reach. The canter must be smooth, straight and unhurried, with three distinct beats.

A pleasure horse, by definition, must first and foremost be cooperative, willing, smooth gaited and well mannered. In addition, some English Pleasure horse classes emphasize brilliance of performance and presence. Brilliance of performance relates to the cadence, expression and degree of flexion and collection of the performance.

In contrast to long, low hunter movement, English Pleasure horses should move with more elevation and animation. The hindquarters should provide the impulsion and power necessary to allow the forehand to be light and airy. The shoulder should exhibit free action, allowing the forearm to reach and lift with a floating motion. This should be accompanied by powerful and well-raised hock action.

A talented English Pleasure horse with uphill conformation (withers higher than the hips) will show these characteristics naturally, and a good trainer will develop the horse and encourage it to express the movement. Shoeing should not be looked at as a means to *make* an English Pleasure horse. However, responsible, conscientious shoeing may enhance performance and prevent the hooves from developing a configuration that might discourage the desired style of movement.

English Pleasure horses often have more upright pasterns, and the hooves should be maintained to align with the pasterns. To elevate

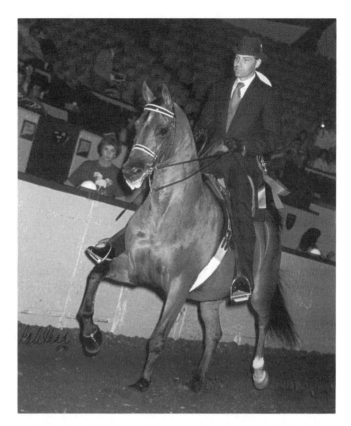

*English Pleasure Horse. Chip Capobianco on Kamma,
Hidden Hill Arabians.* Photo: Robert S. Hess

the horse's forehand and to aid the horse to bringing his knees higher, the front hooves are left longer than normal (and longer than the hinds) and a heavier shoe is applied.

Some associations set limits on the weight of the horseshoe, the thickness of the pad and the total length of the hoof + pad + shoe combination. This effectively restricts the amount of "help" that a horse can be given by shoeing. For example, the shoe weight might be limited to 14 ounces, the maximum pad thickness might be ⅜ inch and the maximum total length (hoof/pad/shoe length = the distance from the coronary rim to the ground surface of the shoe) might be 4½ inches.

A 14-ounce shoe would probably be about ⅜ inch thick. If a ⅜-inch pad is used, then the maximum length the bare trimmed hoof can be is about 3¾ inches—that is, on show day. So, at time of shoeing, the bare hoof would have to be a little bit shorter (⅛ to ⅜ inch depending on individual growth and the amount of time before the show) to allow for normal hoof growth. (By comparison, if the same hoof was shod as a hunter, the bare hoof length would be between 3¼ and 3½ inches.)

If a bar shoe is needed to support the hoof, even with the extra steel that is needed to make the bar, the weight limit cannot be exceeded. As with the hunter shoe, the inside edge of the ground surface of the shoe can be ground out to reduce the weight of the shoe, if necessary. Some show rules prohibit the bar from extending below the ground surface of the shoe.

To make a heavier shoe, the farrier can use steel that is thicker (⅜ inch) than a normal shoe (¼ inch), rather than using a wider shoe. The thicker steel provides more of the total length of the hoof/pad/ shoe, and keeping the web of the shoe narrow maintains traction that would be diminished with a wider web. A lighter shoe is often used when beginning training or at the start of the season.

One thing to bear in mind is that with a longer hoof the breakover point is moved forward and will be further from the center of the hoof (Chapter 5). Therefore, the heels of the shoe are extended to lengthen the base of support and to keep the base centered beneath the hoof. Also, it is common to roll the toes of the front shoes (as much as half the width of the web), which helps ease the increased strain of break- over resulting from the longer toe. Rolling the toes also enhances the action of the limb.

While the forelimbs are shod for elevation, the hind limbs are shod to shift the weight back over the hindquarters. This is done by trim- ming the hind hooves as short as is practical. To accommodate the rearward weight shift, the heels of the hind shoes are often extended or trailered to provide a larger base of support. Some believe that using lateral trailers increases the action of the hinds and helps the horse negotiate turns more confidently. A full-rim shoe is commonly used on the hinds to provide traction. In addition, the toes of the hind shoes are routinely squared to enhance the action, to lessen the chance of a front shoe being stepped off and to prevent the "clicking" sound of forging.

Because the breeds of horses used for English Pleasure often have more upright, solid hooves, clips are not usually required to secure the shoe (and pad) or to maintain hoof shape. If pads are used, they are often leather, which "seats" around the edge of the hoof wall and locks in place. Also popular is a synthetic pad that is manufactured to the maximum legal thickness and has a textured surface designed to prevent the pad from sliding on the hoof surface.

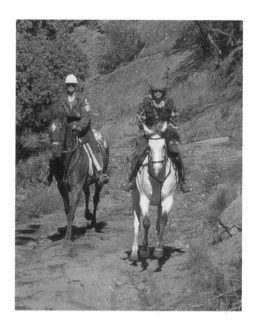

*Long-distance horses. Tawny,
ridden by Jas McMahon, and
Lancer, ridden by Sue Dixon*

LONG-DISTANCE HORSES

Endurance and competitive trail horses (although scored differently in competition) are ridden for long hours and many miles. Because of this, attention to the special shoeing requirements of long-distance horses is critical. Distance shoeing must safeguard soundness, support leg structures and tendons, minimize fatigue, protect the heels and soles and provide adequate traction and wear. The footing long-distance horses might encounter in one shoeing period can include rock, shale, mud, water, gravel, blacktop, hard-pack road, grasslands, sand and snow. The terrain might be level but covered with hummocks and holes, or it might be steeply sloped either uphill or downhill. Therefore, to suit a variety of conditions, most long-distance horses do best simply with plain or rim shoes applied to balanced hooves.

Support Shoes should help to support the distance horse as his muscles tire. The more fatigued a horse is, the more his muscles will "give," increasing the chance of strained tendons and ligaments. This is especially true in the case of a misstep. If the heels of the shoes are long enough so that they are directly below (or even behind) the midpoint of the cannon bone, the horse will likely receive necessary support.

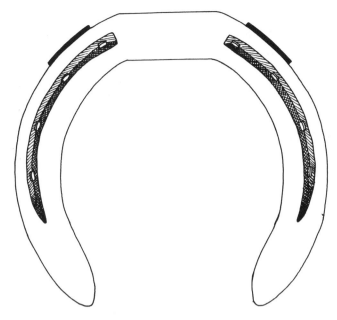

Squared-toe shoe with forward placed side clips

The high-mile horse's shoes should be designed so that minimal energy is required for breakover. The goal is to make breakover as effortless for the muscles and tendons as possible, thereby reducing fatigue, maximizing performance and minimizing the possibility of strain (Chapters 6, 7 and 9).

It is particularly important to provide generous room for normal hoof expansion. With each stride, the weight of the horse (and rider and tack) is sent down to the hooves with an additional force directly proportional to the gait and speed. In order to dissipate this shock effectively, the hoof must be free to deform and re-form, spread at the quarters and then return.

Correct, current shoeing can prevent the development of gait defects. The best of endurance horses might tend to forge when tired. Long-distance riding is predominated by long-legged Arabian and Arabian crossbreds, and these horses often have short backs. In addition, when a rider wants to cover the miles, the goal is distance, not collection, so the horse is often allowed to travel in an extended frame and on its forehand. Fortunately, by balancing the hooves and easing breakover with squared-toe shoes, fatigue and the tendency to forge can be lessened.

Protection One of the primary reasons for shoeing any active horse is to protect the hoof from abrasion—the wall simply wears away faster than it grows. With trail horses, the bulbs of the heels, particularly on the hinds, may be bruised when a horse is scrambling up or sliding down a steep incline. If the heels of the shoe extend adequately, they will help prevent the bulbs from being damaged by the ground. Also, shoes elevate the sole from the ground and help prevent bruising of the sole and frog.

Pads are sometimes used for added protection. Rim pads will put more space between the sole and the ground, and some might absorb a degree of concussion. However, tubular rim pads do not hold up well on the high-mile horse. Full pads protect and wear better but result in a heavier hoof and decreased traction, major considerations with endurance horses (Chapters 4 and 6).

Traction The traction required by a distance horse is usually adequately provided by a plain steel shoe. If desired, more traction can be obtained by using a rim shoe. Aggressive traction devices, such as studs, toe or heel calks or excess borium height should be avoided, as too much grab can result in wrenched ligaments. Borium applied thinly and evenly on the toes and heels of the shoes might be helpful during slippery weather. During winter months, borium-headed nails or short (¼ inch) studs will provide a little more bite if it is necessary to train on frozen ground (Chapter 4). Normally during the competition season, however, trail conditions do not require the addition of any traction devices.

Wear Long-distance horses, in general, have healthy hooves and vigorous hoof growth because of good nutrition and adequate exercise. Therefore, there is usually little difficulty finding solid new hoof to nail to every six weeks. Farrier appointments should be scheduled carefully in relation to the dates of upcoming races. Ideally, a horse should have new shoes about seven to ten days before a race.

Even during the pre-competition conditioning season, when the horse is covering the most miles, a set of normal steel shoes usually will last five or six weeks. But if a horse is routinely conditioned on hard roads or rocky terrain, fine grit borium or a hard surfacing material may need to be added to increase its wear resistance.

Synthetic hoof boots have been used in lieu of and in combination with shoes. A set of boots will last about two hundred miles; their life can be extended by inserting a layer of sorbothane between the shoe and the boot. It is always advisable to carry a rubber boot of the appropriate size along on rides in case of a lost shoe (see Resource Guide in the Appendix). Also, it is a good idea to have your regular farrier shape an extra set of shoes for you to take to competitions so that if your horse loses a shoe, it can be replaced with the appropriate shoe.

REINING

The precision maneuvers at high speeds that a reining horse performs requires balanced, *preventive* shoeing coupled with some specialized shoeing techniques. Starting from a standstill, the reining horse is often required to lope with increasing speed until he is running flat out. In a delicate balance, the thundering energy of the run is transformed into a smooth, deep stop. As the forehand elevates and the hind end melts into the ground, the residual power of the run sends the horse sliding forward thirty feet or more while the front legs march alternately in a smooth cadence.

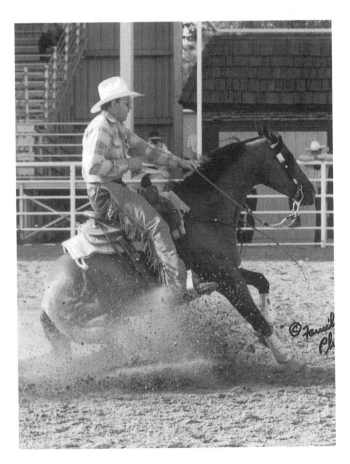

Sliding stop performed by Les Vogt on Chex A Nic, 1992 AQHA and NRCHA World Champion. Photo: Jim Clanin, Family Photos

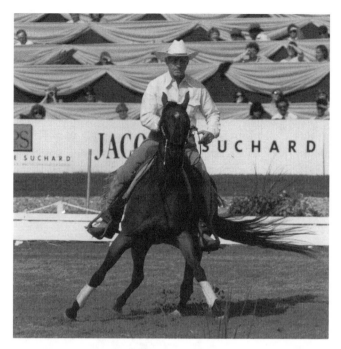

Turnaround by Alotalena,
with Dick Pieper riding.
Photo: Valerie Parry

In the turnaround, the horse's body whirls around the inside hind foot as the front legs reach and cross over in a precise but smooth motion. When turning to the left, the right front leg crosses in front of and past the left front leg, then the left front leg reaches out from behind and steps wide to the left. The pattern repeats with rapid fire. Just a slight imbalance can create the potential for bone bruises, fractured splint bones or coronary injuries. Therefore, a balanced hoof is essential. Conformation, talent and training play the largest parts in a reining horse's performance. The role of shoeing is to help maintain soundness and to allow the horse to perform in a balanced and secure fashion.

It is no surprise that when a horse is asked to move with a high degree of speed and lateral movement that he lands on one side of his hoof with more impact. A horse actually drives with the side of his hoof in the spin. High quarter cracks, originating at the coronary band on either the medial or lateral side, occur fairly frequently with reining horses. These cracks are often due to interference from a misstep during training. Proper training starts with balanced, correct form. Then speed is added. If the horse is asked to spin fast before

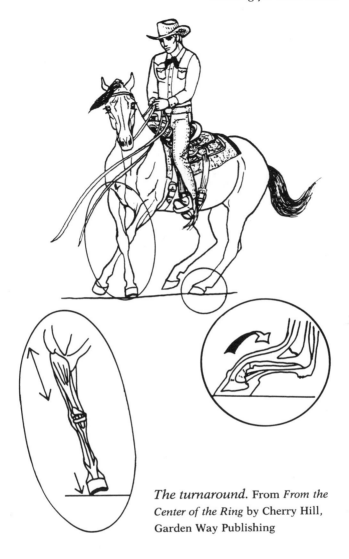

The turnaround. From *From the Center of the Ring* by Cherry Hill, Garden Way Publishing

he is ready, he may step on or hit the coronary band and bruise it. The weakened area is then vulnerable and often forms a horizontal crack at the coronary band called a blow-out crack (Chapter 11). Especially if the hoof is imbalanced, such a defect in the hoof can develop into a quarter crack that extends toward the ground surface.

The best defense against these cracks is to not push a horse too fast in its training, to use protective bell boots (see Resource Guide in the Appendix), to carefully monitor hoof balance and to develop and maintain the strongest hoof structure possible. Hoof tissues need to be conditioned just as bone and muscle tissues do before they reach their optimum strength.

Rinsing a horse daily after workouts begins a stressful wet/dry cycle that can predispose hooves to cracking. Applying a hoof sealer (see Resource Guide in the Appendix) to help stabilize the hoof moisture may be helpful as well as feeding a supplement formulated specifically for development of sound hoof tissues (see Resource Guide in the Appendix).

Half-round shoes are sometimes used on the front feet of a reining horse so he can easily break over in any direction and spin flatter or lower to the ground. Since pivots and turnarounds require so much lateral movement, these shoes make the mechanics of the job easier for the hoof. However, some trainers and shoers don't feel that a standard half-round has a web wide enough to give the front feet the support they require for the amount of galloping in a reining horse's training and conditioning program. And a half-round shoe that is wide enough for support is so heavy that it can cause exaggerated action. The rounded edges of polo or rim shoes (Chapter 6) serve the

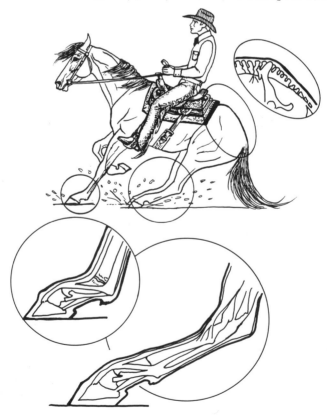

The sliding stop. From *From the Center of the Ring* by Cherry Hill, Garden Way Publishing

same purpose of the half-round and are usually wider webbed and lighter, and provide traction. Wide-web aluminum shoes with beveled edges are also used.

During the rundown, stop and turnaround, the reining horse experiences hyperextension of his fetlock joints. As the ergots come close to or touch the ground, the flexor muscles and tendons have stretched to near capacity. To provide the support necessary for these maneuvers, the heels of the front shoes must meet the support criteria for preventive shoeing as described in Chapter 5.

Many reining horses really like performing sliding stops. Good footing and proper shoeing can make a horse's job easier and less stressful. Sliding plates are usually hand made by the farrier from ¾ to 1¼ inches wide by ¼ inch flat bar stock. The shoes have characteristic extended heels called trailers, which increase surface area and add to the horse's support, stability and balance. The trailers seldom extend past the bulbs of the heel. Extremely long trailers can cut the opposite leg during the turnaround.

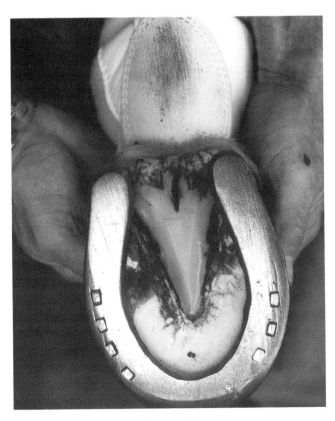

Sliding plate

The nail heads of sliders are countersunk and filed off flush with the shoe if necessary after they are nailed to the horse's hoof. This very smooth ground surface reduces friction so the horse can glide to his stop. The inside edge of the ground surface of the sliding plate is beveled to prevent dirt from packing in the sole area. To reduce friction even more during the stop, the ground surface of the toe of a sliding plate can be tapered from credit-card thin at the top of the toe to the full ¼-inch thickness at the back of the toe. This will allow the slider to act more like a ski than a plow. Of course, this tapered shoe will wear out faster and need to be replaced more frequently. Sliders don't *teach* a horse how to stop, but they can make it easier for him to do the right thing. Sliding plates also help minimize the stressful effects of torque in the turnaround. The smooth surface of the shoe allows the pivot foot to swivel in its position and provides a big, wide base for lateral support.

Clips may be used with sliders on weak hooves to counteract the forces that tend to shift the shoe backwards. This takes much strain off the nails. Once nails get loose and movement begins, the hoof wall can split and break.

As a young horse is learning to add speed to his turnaround, he may tend to step on the inside branch of his slider and pull it off. So sometimes as a temporary measure when the horse is going through this stage, the inside trailer might be left a little shorter.

Because a sliding plate is an anti-traction shoe, if the width of the shoe that is used is extreme, a horse might slip when loping circles. In most cases, 1-inch sliding plates with equal length branches provide adequate traction for all components of the reining pattern on most competition footings. If a horse needs a little help developing his stop, sliders that are 1¼ inches wide at the toe and taper to ¾ inch at the heel are sometimes used. A sliding plate 1¼ inches wide throughout the shoe would be too slippery, and the weight would cause a horse to snap his hocks.

Horses that run with a long stride have the potential of reaching forward with their hind legs and pulling off their front shoes. With a hard, deep stopper, there is also the possibility of the front shoes being pulled when the horse first goes to the ground with his hind legs as they reach deep under his abdomen.

Some horses (often in their three-year-old year) go through a phase of losing shoes during their training. This often occurs because the horse is still learning the precise timing required for a balanced stop (Chapter 7). Rather than beginning to stop by bending at the loin when the leading foreleg is on the ground as a seasoned reiner does, the young horse might react to the trainer's signal out of sync and start to stop at the wrong moment of his lope stride, such as when the diagonal pair is on the ground. The result? He plucks off a front shoe.

If a horse has a tendency to lose front shoes, it is tempting to shorten the heels of the front shoes to prevent them from being stepped off. But this will only shorten the support base of the front limbs and set the horse up for injuries to the tendons and ligaments. Giving the horse even more support with a longer heel (if the farrier has the courage to try it) actually helps *prevent* lost shoes because the heel doesn't sink into the footing so far, therefore it takes less time and effort for the hoof to spring off the ground and break over. Modifying the toes of the front shoes (Chapter 6) can also help speed the breakover of the front hoof just enough to get them out of the hind's way. The best thing to do when a horse loses a shoe is to put it back on, and put it on in such a manner that if it is stepped off it comes off clean and doesn't take a large portion of hoof with it.

For long-term soundness, it is best to shoe a reining horse following principles of preventive shoeing. Sometimes, in an attempt to get a horse to slide straight, without his hind legs spreading, the sliders are positioned on the hoof so that even if the hooves point outward the shoes are pointing straight ahead. However, this can result in a horse with sore hocks and stifles.

Other harmful "tricks" used to straighten a slide include trimming the hind hooves imbalanced to one side, using an inside grab on the slider or bending the inside trailer down toward the ground, all of which put uneven stress on the hoof and limb and can lead to sheared heels and serious joint problems. Leaving the toes of the hind hooves extremely long and with a low hoof angle and applying very long, wide sliders that cover most of the bottom of the hoof are also misguided methods of "helping" the horse to slide. The fact is, the most talented reining horse in the world cannot compete successfully if he is not sound. The development of a top reining horse has more to do with conformation, preventive shoeing and solid training than it does with shoeing gimmicks that jeopardize the horse's soundness. If a horse is conscientiously trained for reining and cannot do the job, he should be used for a different event rather than having his performance drastically altered by shoeing.

CUTTING AND WORKING COW HORSE

The cutting horse must enter a herd of cattle and, with help from his rider, cut an animal out of the herd and drive it away from the herd. Once the cow is isolated near the center of the arena and away from the herd, the rider discontinues his cues to the horse and allows the horse to display his inherent cow sense, his natural physical agility and the thoroughness of his training. The cutting horse must react instantly to a cow's every move to prevent the cow from returning to the herd. This results in some seemingly impossible movements at high speed as the horse pounces back and forth like a savvy cat.

The working cow horse must perform a reining pattern and cow work. The cow work includes the horse controlling the cow by holding it at the end of the arena as well as confining it in a tight circle. The horse must also turn the cow along a fence, which requires the horse to run at full speed to catch and pass the cow, then stop, turn into the cow and be ready to run at full speed in the opposite direction. The shoeing of the working cow horse requires a combination of reining and cutting shoeing techniques. Shoeing the hinds moderately (with ¾-inch sliders) allows the working cow horse to perform the reining pattern, yet prevents him from sliding past the cow on the fence or slipping when he circles the cow.

To allow the cutting horse or cow horse to move as freely as possible, he would be shod as naturally as possible. Close attention

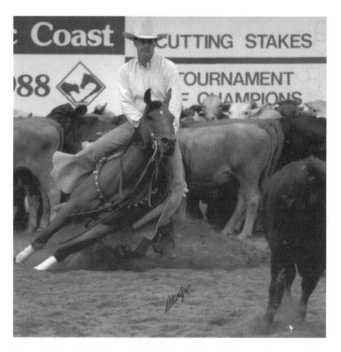

Ima Thirsty Oak, with Al Dunning riding. Photo: Midge Ames

should be paid to maintaining a short hoof length and keeping the hoof in proper DP and ML balance. Any dish at the toe should be controlled to keep the base of support back under the leg.

As with other events, the more comfortable the cutting or cow horse is, the more trainable he will be and the better he will perform. If a cutting horse has underrun heels, he can be made more comfortable with a longer shoe or an egg bar shoe. If his heels are low, they can be raised temporarily with a bar wedge pad or wedge shoe. The short-term risk of a lost shoe is more than offset by the long-term benefits of shoeing a cutting horse for soundness. If a good measure of support is given to the front feet by generous heel length, the horse will not rock back into the footing, and he will get more lift coming out of the ground. The front shoes are often rockered or rolled to help the horse break over quicker.

Because of the extreme quickness, change of direction and close movement of the limbs, some farriers are tempted to fit the shoe very close, eliminating the normal room for expansion. This lessens the chance that the horse will step off a shoe. But without the expansion room, the hoof will often spread beyond the shoe and "drop down" over the shoe, damaging the hoof horn at the heels, which will result in a low angle. If the expansion room of the shoe is compromised, it is important that the shoes are reset more frequently to prevent the hoof spreading over the edge of the shoes.

The quick maneuvers the cutting horse performs require good traction, but too much traction will interfere with the natural flow and grace of the movements. Calks are rarely used because of the strain they put on the leg structures. Likewise, trailers are avoided because of the chance of interfering and injuring the opposite limb.

Many top cutting horses perform well in plain steel shoes. Others require the extra traction of a rim shoe. In some cases a rim shoe might provide too much grab, so a plain aluminum shoe is used to provide a gentle grip. Side clips are used, especially on the hinds, to keep the shoes in place during the strenuous lateral movements.

SPEED EVENTS AND ROPING

Barrel racing, pole bending and the keyhole race are three of the most common speed events. Calf roping, team roping and steer wrestling (aka bulldogging) are three of the most popular timed cattle events. In all of these classes, the fastest horse and rider team to properly complete their job wins.

A roping horse must burst out of the roping box to catch a calf or steer that has about a 20-foot head start. The horse runs at full speed then must stop instantly and hard, with no extended sliding like a reining horse. In team roping, the heading horse must also "log" the 550-pound steer, that is, slow him down and hold him in position so the heeler can catch him. The calf-roping horse has a specialized aspect to his performance, too. He must "run backward" to take the slack out of the rope once the 350-pound calf is caught. Winning times in roping are often separated by a hundredth of a second.

A barrel racing horse runs around three barrels in a cloverleaf pattern at full speed. This requires the horse to make tight turns in both directions with balance. Because of very close times, some competitions utilize electronic timers that give the score in thousandths of a second.

Because of the quick turns and tremendous bursts of speed required in these timed events, the horses can easily lose shoes. It is best to begin by shoeing with the optimum size shoe, leaving normal expansion room of about ⅛ inch and normal heel extension. Many horses perform fine under these guidelines without losing shoes. In fact, some roping and barrel horses routinely wear egg bar or extended heel shoes, but other horses tend to lose a shoe with any extra heel length.

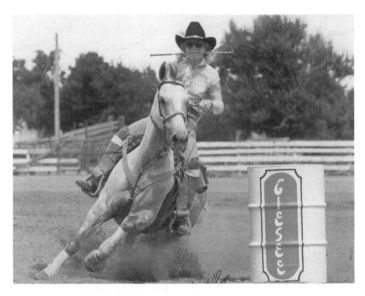

Barrel Racing. Lynn Brown on I Am Clipt. Photo: Hubbell Rodeo Photos

If front shoes are being stepped off, adjustments can be made that will not compromise the support base: using bell boots, spooning the heels of the front shoes, using heel shields on the fronts (Chapter 15), squaring the toes of the hind and/or front shoes and rounding the edges of the shoe on both the hoof surface and the ground surface (see figure on page 32) are all procedures that will not sacrifice support or expansion.

If these adjustments do not solve the problem of lost shoes, then it may be necessary to compromise a bit by shortening the shoe heels and fitting the shoe a little closer at the quarters. (The closer the shoe is fit, the more often the shoes must be reset to prevent the hoof from spreading over the shoe and damaging the heels of the hoof.) There is seldom justification for shortening the heels of the hind shoes. If the shoes are shifting on the hooves, side clips will help to lock them in place.

Roping horses are often shod on the fronts with plain or rim shoes. The hinds are shod, with plain shoes having extended heels. When the horse comes to a sudden stop, it is necessary for his hind feet to slide to some extent. That is why rim shoes or calks are seldom used on the hinds. The extended heels provide support during the stop and also protect the heel bulbs from rough footing. If the hind shoes need squared toes, the front edge of the shoe should be rolled to prevent it from digging in during the stop, which could cause the horse's hind end to hop. The calf horse can sometimes be helped to move backward more smoothly by spooning the heels of the hind shoes, which prevents them from digging into the arena footing.

Barrel racing requires a light shoe that provides support and traction. Most often a rim shoe, a light rim shoe or a polo shoe is used on the front. The rim shoe is slightly heavier than the other two, but it will give the hoof more support (fractures of the coffin bone are common in barrel horses). The polo shoe is the lightest of the three, and the high inside rim gives good traction while the rounded edges let the hoof break over in any direction. The lighter shoes are more appropriate on strong, upright hooves that can get by with less support. Aluminum is sometimes used.

The hinds of barrel horses are shod with either a rim shoe or a plain shoe. A plain shoe will allow the horse to slide into the turns without hopping. If the hind shoes are tapped and threaded, short calks can be added to provide more traction if necessary for different arenas (Chapter 4 and Jumping in this chapter).

Since speed and roping horses perform in many different arenas during the season, often far from the regular farrier, it is a good idea to take along an extra set of shoes, shaped and ready to go on. Also, many of these horses perform best one or two weeks into their shoeing period, so strategic scheduling of farrier appointments will help optimize performance throughout the season.

POLO

Few events place greater demands on the horse than does polo. Levels of polo are defined by the ability of the players and their horses. Players are rated on a scale of 1 to 10 goals. Although high-goal polo is what is covered in magazines and/or television, most players have a rating of 2 goals or less. Polo is played almost entirely at a gallop, which is why each player rides two to eight different horses in each game. Horses must be able to change direction at a gallop. This fast-paced contact sport places great stress on a horse's body and legs, consequently shoeing must provide traction yet meet the requirements of the United States Polo Association (USPA).

Certain types of shoes and traction devices are outlawed by the USPA to prevent horses from cutting each other during close contact. The polo shoe has a higher inside rim that provides traction on most playing fields. It is also lightweight and allows easy breakover in all directions. The polo shoe is used almost exclusively on the front feet, although if a horse has a poor-quality hoof needing more support, a heavier rim shoe can be used. Polo horses that play indoors do not require the traction of a polo shoe, so are often shod with a light version of the rim shoe.

The front toes of the polo horse are kept short and at a natural or slightly steeper angle to facilitate agility and cut down on fatigue. Long toe/low heel (Chapter 11) would be very hard on a polo horse's limbs. The hind toes are kept short for the same reasons and to minimize overreaching and lost shoes.

Because of the extreme force put on the hooves of a polo horse when turning quickly at high speeds, traction should be monitored with great discretion (Chapter 4). If the horse requires more traction than provided by a rim shoe or a polo shoe, the hinds can be shod with a plain steel shoe with forged dull heel calks. The calks should be forged on both heels to provide maximum traction. Borium is considered a sharp calk and is prohibited.

Instead of side clips, toe clips are often used to keep the calked shoe from sliding back on the hoof. Side clips lock the shoe onto the hoof very securely, and if the shoe gets a good bite in the turf, it is better for the horse to slide off the shoe than to risk a fracture of the pastern. On the other hand, a shoe with less traction that *is* secured by side clips not only lessens the risk of a fracture but also avoids the damage to the hoof wall that often occurs with a lost shoe. Trailers are seldom used on polo horses because of the danger of another horse stepping on them.

JUMPING AND CROSS COUNTRY

Jumper fences are more colorful and unusual, higher and wider than hunter fences. Jumping lines on the course are usually tricky, meeting the fences at sharp angles and requiring hard turns. Jumper classes are scored on faults and often on time. Therefore, the jumper must be aggressive, powerful and agile. Cross country is a phase of eventing that involves jumping more "natural" obstacles on a large, open course. Shoeing is an important part of a jumping horse's confidence formula. And traction is one of the key elements in that formula (Chapters 4 and 6).

Screw-in calks (studs) are threaded so they can be removed or changed according to the phase of an event or the footing. Drive-in calks have a smooth, tapered shaft that fits tightly into a hole in the shoe. Studs usually have bullet-shaped or blocky heads and range in height from $1\frac{1}{16}$ inch for show jumpers to $\frac{1}{2}$-inch road calks. Although removable studs offer the advantage of applying the right amount of traction for a particular footing, the sudden change may not allow a horse to adapt to his new traction. Studs should not be used on narrow-web shoes because the hole that is required will weaken the shoe and it could break. Your farrier must drill for drive-in studs and tap (make threads) for screw-in studs after the shoe has been shaped for the hoof.

To put a stud into a tapped shoe, rotate a slender screwdriver in the hole to remove the dirt. Then spray a strong stream of penetrating oil into the hole to flush out the rest of the dirt and lubricate the threads. Use a thread-cleaning tool to carefully clean the rest of the dirt out. Then screw in the stud, being sure it is securely tightened with a wrench.

Calks should be removed whenever the horse is not being used so the horse does not injure himself. The hole in the shoe can either be left open to pack with dirt or filled with a screw-in flush metal plug. However, screw-in plugs often get damaged with wear and can be difficult to remove. Petroleum jelly or oil and cotton packed weekly or a piece of small rubber tubing can act as a plug and protect the threads. However, these too can be difficult to remove. Often letting

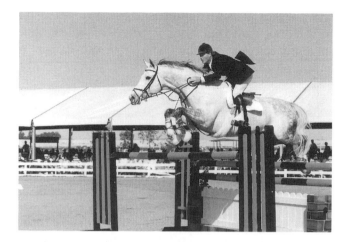

Grand Prix jumper Arthos, with John McConnell riding. Photo: Tish Quick, courtesy of Patty Arnette

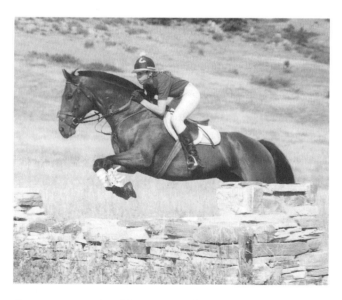

Cross country. Kathleen Donnelly riding. From *Becoming an Effective Rider,* by Cherry Hill, Garden Way Publishing

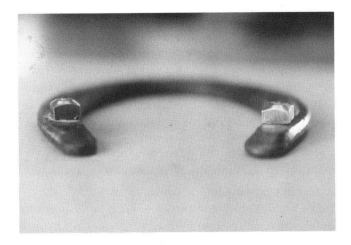

Short screw-in studs

the hole fill with dirt is the easiest option. Removing the accumulated dirt can be made easier by packing the holes with wax (see Resource Guide in the Appendix) each time the studs are removed.

There are many choices of studs in terms of shape of head, height and thread size. The most conservative is a dip stud, which is a drive-in plug that fits flush with the shoe, allowing just the tungsten center pin to protrude $\frac{1}{16}$ inch above the shoe. Threaded studs tend to have blocky or bullet-shaped heads and range in height from the $\frac{1}{4}$-inch (above the shoe) "road calks" to the $1\frac{1}{16}$-inch studs for show jumpers. Although studs are available in various thread sizes, the standard is $\frac{3}{8}$ inch.

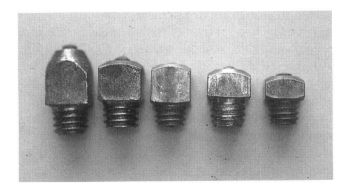

Stud assortment

Some of the more popular studs are Mordax RS, B, Olympic and Stromsholm grass studs TSL and TSH (see Resource Guide in the Appendix). Some jumper and event riders keep a selection of calks on hand for a variety of conditions and put the appropriate ones in just before their round. Usually larger calks are applied to the hinds than the fronts. It is popular to use three studs on a hind shoe, one at each heel and the third placed on the outside branch between the third and fourth nails. This gives the horse a little more grab on the turns. Because today's calks have a tungsten carbide center pin, the calks start out "soft" and round, and as they wear they become "sharp," due to the emerging point at the center.

Jar calks, which are more commonly seen on hunters than jumpers, are rectangular or triangular pieces of steel that are brazed on the shoes to prevent sideways slipping while allowing the hoof to slide forward on landing. They are usually applied at the heels and set in the direction of travel, not parallel to the angled heels of the shoe. However, if the goal is to decrease both sideways and forward/backward slipping, the jar calks can be placed parallel to the heels of the shoe. It is advisable that clips be used with calks.

SHOEING FOR THE STREETS: POLICE AND PARADE HORSES

The hard surface of most city streets is rigid and unyielding. Therefore, it is essential that street horses are shod to land flat or comfort and soundness are compromised and hoof imbalance problems such as sheared heels, displaced coronet or cracks could occur (Chapter 11).

The street horse's traction requirements coupled with the excessive wear from working on pavement present a unique shoeing situation. Options include steel shoes with studs or borium, rubber shoes over a steel core and plastic shoes over a steel or aluminum core. (All plastic nail-on shoes do not provide the hoof with sufficient support.) Plastic and rubber shoes (with metal cores) work well on clean dry pavement but are dangerously slippery if there is sand or dirt on the street or if the road is wet. Both plastic and rubber shoes are very slippery on grass. Rubber shoes provide good shock absorption but are bulky and difficult to shape. Studs direct focal pressure to the hoof where the studs are located and can cause bruising. Studs also tear up the road surface.

Therefore, the best option is borium on steel shoes with clips and

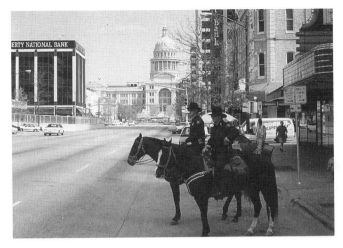

Austin Mounted Police Officers Russ Jensen and Mike Carlson

rim pads. A horse should be started with fine-grit borium (small particles of tungsten) until he learns to handle himself on pavement. Increasingly courser borium (larger particles of tungsten) can be added at subsequent shoeings to provide more grab. Using a wide-web shoe allows the borium to be applied along the inside of the web so borium will not contact the horse and cut him if he steps on himself.

Since police horses are regularly worked on hard surfaces a shock-absorbing rim pad (either a tube-type rim pad or a flat rubber rim pad) is used to ensure soundness. It has been found that trimming the hooves of street horses slightly steeper than normal (so that the hoof appears to have a broken forward hoof/pastern axis) adds to their comfort and long-term soundness.

WINTER RIDING

No matter what your event, if you ride outdoors in a temperate climate in the winter, your horse will have some special shoeing needs. One approach is to have your horse's shoes pulled for the winter (Chapter 4). At the other end of the spectrum is having your equine athlete shod with pads and studs so he can train in all types of footing.

To design your winter hoof care program, consider the natural conformation of your horse's hooves, the level and type of his exercise during the winter months, the footing in his exercise and turnout areas, the typical weather patterns in your locale and the expertise of your farrier.

The barefoot horse with a naturally balanced hoof, dense hoof horn and a well-cupped sole is often able to grip many winter footings without hoof damage. And a naturally concave sole sheds snow, mud and slush well. However, a hoof with a long toe and low heel, brittle or punky horn and a flat sole has poor traction, and the sole is vulnerable to bruising from frozen ground. During the winter, the hoof growth rate can slow to almost half its spring rate; that means the hoof cannot stand a great deal of abrasive wear. Therefore, for active winter riding, a horse should be shod. Shoeing offers protection for the hoof and helps to maintain proper balance. In addition, winter shoeing can serve two other purposes: providing additional traction and preventing snowballing.

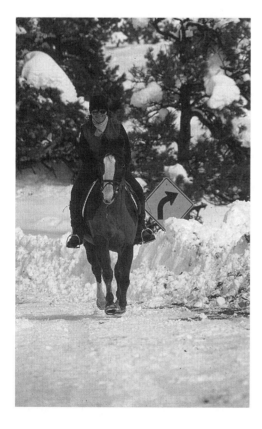

Winter shoes allow Cherry Hill to enjoy a ride on Zinger

Traction

Various amounts of traction are available depending on the techniques used by your farrier (Chapter 4 and Jumping in this chapter). Rim shoes provide more traction than plain shoes, and aluminum shoes have a slightly better grab on frozen ground because the metal is softer. Aluminum racing plates with toe grabs and/or heel stickers could be appropriate for moderate work in relatively soft footing. Rubber and plastic shoes tend to provide less traction than either the bare hoof or steel shoes and are hard and slippery in cold weather.

Steel keg shoes with permanent calks forged at the toe and/or heels sink into semifrozen ground or "soft" ice and give good traction. However, on hard ice such shoes are dangerously slippery. Removable studs allow for adaptation to the constantly changing winter footing conditions.

A hard surfacing material such as borium can be applied at the toe and/or heel of the horse's regular steel or aluminum shoes in smears, beads or points. A torch or forge is used to melt the carrier metal and adhere carbide grit or chips of various sizes to the shoe surface. Borium works best when used at a ⅛- to ¼-inch thickness.

Very effective winter traction devices can be made by applying borium to the heads of ³⁄₁₆- by ⁵⁄₁₆-inch flat rivets. These traction buttons are inserted into holes drilled in front of or behind the last nail hole and are either brazed or welded in place. Two buttons per shoe will provide sufficient traction for most winter conditions.

Nails with ribbed or specially hardened heads can be substituted for regular horseshoe nails to allow a horse to grab onto the ground. The treated heads resist wear and their points dig into ice. The specialized nails are installed at the midpoint (third or fourth nail holes) of the hoof. This provides optimum traction without adversely affecting the landing or breakover. Usually two nails are used per shoe.

Extreme ice nail height is an added danger for both horses and humans in the event of a kick or a misstep. And although they do provide good traction in snow or soft ice, when the horse is moving on uneven frozen ground, commercial ice nails can provide too much stick and torque, which may lead to leg problems.

Anti-Snowballing

When mixtures of snow, ice, mud, manure, grass or bedding accumulate in the sole area, it can pack densely into large rounded ice mounds that are almost impossible to chip out. The junction of the inner edge of the shoe with the sole provides a place for the mud and ice to become securely lodged. Snow will melt from the heat of the sole and freeze onto the metal horseshoe, and the snowball will begin. When a horse is forced to stand or move on the snowballs, he has decreased stability in his fetlock joint. His weight is liable to suddenly roll medially, laterally, forward or backward. It is extremely fatiguing for his muscles, tendons and joint ligaments, as he constantly must make adjustments to maintain his equilibrium. It is easy for a snowballed horse to momentarily lose his balance and wrench a fetlock.

Applying various substances such as grease to the sole of the barefoot or shod horse or spraying it with a nonstick cooking coating may prevent snow buildup during certain temperatures, but only temporarily. Half-round shoes do a fair job of shedding snow because of the inside rounded edge. However, half-rounds provide poor winter traction, so ice nails or borium should be used with them.

Full pads can help prevent snowballing in some situations. The choices include plastic, synthetic rubber, sorbothane and leather (listed in the order of their ability to resist snow buildup). Full pads with a convex bubble at the sole seem to be only marginally better than full flat pads at popping out accumulated snow. Traction is decreased with full pads.

Tube-type rim pads (See Resource Guide in the Appendix) that fit

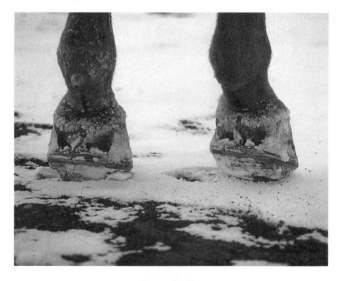

Snowballs

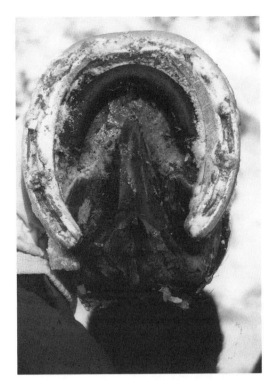

Winter shoes

between the shoe and the hoof wall leaving the sole open are the best anti-snowballing option. The sole retains its cupped traction feature, can respire normally and can descend with weight bearing. As the horse's weight descends on the hoof, the pads flex and dislodge the snow that accumulates at the junction of the shoe and sole. Tube pads with open shoes work well in most weather conditions. Bar shoes (egg bar shoes, full support shoes, etc.) will trap snow and not allow the tube pads to do their job as effectively.

There are combinations of snow type and temperature where it is impossible to provide safe traction and prevent snowballing. However, in most types of winter footing, good results can be obtained by a combination of the horse's normal shoes with an application of various traction and anti-snowballing devices.

Common Problems

Hoof, foot and limb problems hinder a horse's performance. Identifying and treating problems early often prevents permanent damage. Remember, shoeing is just one part of the sound horse formula. Provide your horses with the highest level of management and training possible, and work closely with your farrier and veterinarian when solving problems. For a thorough coverage of lameness, refer to the Recommended Reading list in the Appendix.

NEGLECT

Failing to provide regular, competent hoof care is a main cause of problems. Neglect includes allowing the bare foot to wear too short; to grow so long that it breaks off; leaving shoes on so long that the hoof grows over the shoe or grows very imbalanced; overfeeding and underfeeding, and failure to examine the hooves regularly for embedded rocks, nails and other foreign objects.

HOOF DAMAGE

Broken hooves can alter hoof balance and cause lameness (see photograph on page 16). However, it is not uncommon for flared hooves to break yet the horse remain sound. Similarly, a horse can rip off a shoe and portions of hoof wall and be reshod routinely. But when a large section of hoof wall is missing, hoof repair may be necessary.

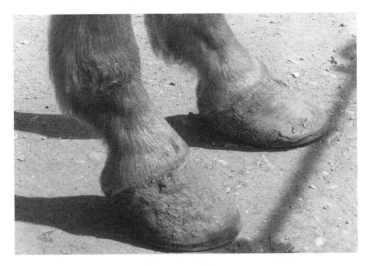

Owner neglect

Your farrier can use hoof repair materials that have properties very similar to hoof horn and will adhere to the hoof wall for months until new growth replaces the damaged area. These materials can be used to build up the low side of a hoof, replace missing sections of wall or build up thin walls so a shoe can be nailed on. The prosthetic hoof can be trimmed and shaped like a normal hoof and is strong enough to secure a nail-on shoe. (See Resource Guide in the Appendix.)

If the hoof wall is too weak or damaged to secure a shoe using nails, or if the horse is in too much pain to allow the driving of nails into the hoof, glue-on shoes are an alternative. These shoes are available in configurations for various applications from foal treatment to racing to founder treatment. One type of glue-on shoe utilizes a cuff to which a steel or aluminum shoe of choice is riveted and the cuff glued or taped to the hoof. Another type has plastic tabs around the edge of the shoe that are glued onto the surface of the hoof wall. (See Resource Guide in the Appendix.)

POOR HOOF QUALITY

Good-quality hoof horn is dry, hard and tough, not brittle, spongy or soft. Poor nutrition, faulty metabolism, unhealthy environment, improper management, disease, certain drugs and trauma are all factors that can affect hoof quality.

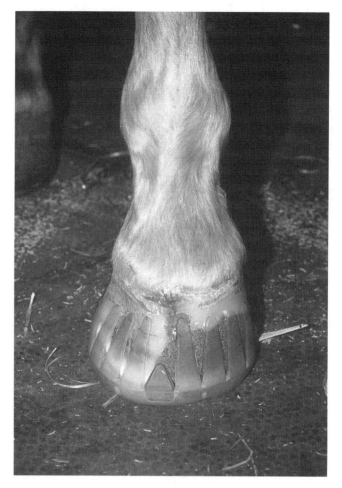

Glue-on shoe

In some cases, poor hoof quality is caused by poor nutrition. In others, the problem lies with the horse's inability to synthesize essential nutrients. A horse's ration should provide adequate amounts of the essential amino acid DL-methionine, biotin (a component of the vitamin B complex) and other nutrients. Often it is necessary to utilize a supplement to meet a horse's nutritional requirements (see Resource Guide in the Appendix). If nutrition is adequate, poor-quality hoofs might be due to other genetic influences and/or poor management practices.

Some horses' feet are so susceptible to excess environmental moisture that daily rinsing or a brief period in mud will cause the wall to weaken. If a hoof suffers from a moisture imbalance, whether it be from a too-wet or too-dry environment, it will usually benefit from regular application of a hoof sealer. Unlike traditional thick or creamy hoof dressings, hoof sealers soak into the hoof wall and remain there to keep external moisture from entering the hoof and internal moisture from evaporating. These sealers are especially useful for hooves covered with tiny surface cracks, which are caused by moisture changes. (See Resource Guide in the Appendix.)

POOR HOOF SHAPE

The hoof capsule is a very plastic structure that adapts in shape to the stresses that are placed upon it. It is more plastic the higher its moisture content. Fortunately, many deformed hooves can be re-formed by the farrier. Every time the hoof is trimmed, its shape should be evaluated and adjusted to assure it is growing in the proper manner. When a hoof is being actively re-formed, the change in shape during one trimming may be dramatic. But even with "normal" feet, with each shoeing the hoof must be shaped and the shoe carefully adjusted. Whether this is done or not is often the difference between a "good" farrier and a "fast" farrier.

Flares in the sidewalls of the hoof can result from ML imbalance, a genetically or nutritionally weak hoof structure, a too-high moisture content in the hoof, or most likely, a combination of these factors. A flare on only one side of the hoof is usually caused by ML

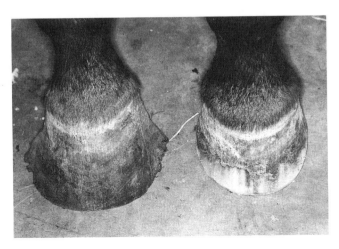

Before and after trimming

imbalance. The flare should be dressed off and that side of the wall should be shortened (lowered). The quarter where the flare was located should be sculpted out with the rasp so the hoof at that area bears no weight. This removes the bending forces on the horn tubules and will result in the new hoof horn growing down straight.

If the hoof wall flares out on both sides, it is usually a combination of hoof conformation and high moisture. Many horses have "pancake" hooves that tend to spread out and become very flat. The treatment for these hooves includes stabilizing their moisture content by keeping them in a dry environment and applying a hoof sealer to minimize the absorption of external moisture. The flares should be dressed off to about half the thickness of the hoof wall and a shoe applied with side clips located across the widest part of the flared hoof (see figure on page 76). (The shoe should be a bar shoe or an open shoe that is strong enough to withstand the spreading forces of the hoof.) The straighter the hoof wall becomes, the stronger it is. Once the shape of the hoof is restored and the moisture content stabilized, the hoof can often be shod with a regular shoe with no clips.

Often the hoof is not flared symmetrically but is distorted across the diagonal of the hoof base, such as a medial toe flare with a lateral heel flare. Along with this, the opposing points (the medial heel and lateral toe) will be pulled inward. Trimming the hoof into balance may prevent further distortion of the hoof, but a shoe is usually required to re-form the hoof to a more functional symmetric shape. The shoe is applied with clips across the longest diagonal. These clips will contain the hoof as it grows down, encouraging expansion across the narrow diagonal, and the result will be a more symmetric hoof.

A flare at the front of the hoof wall is called a dish. Most hooves will dish to some degree, and as part of the regular trimming process this dish should be dressed so the hoof wall at the toe is straight from the coronet to the ground. If this is not done, the dish will cause the breakover point of the hoof and the entire base of support to be too far forward. The presence of any dish can easily be seen by laying a straight edge such as a rasp against the hoof wall.

A dished toe is sometimes the result of a contraction of the muscle-tendon unit at the back of the limb. This contraction exerts constant pull on the coffin bone within the hoof capsule, which causes the hoof wall to bend away from the coffin bone and result in a dish. The treatment is to elevate the angle of the hoof by trimming or by using a wedge pad or shoe. This will often lessen the pull on the coffin bone enough to allow the muscle-tendon unit to relax. Then, if necessary, the hoof may be lowered over several trimming periods back to its normal angle.

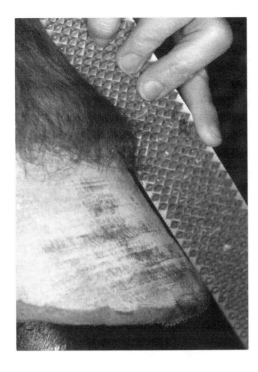

Checking for a dish

A club foot or even just a normally steep hoof might develop a dish if the heels are lowered too much in an attempt to "balance" the foot. These types of hooves are better maintained at a relatively steep angle of 60 to 65 degrees.

As with flares, an increase in hoof moisture will allow the hoof wall to dish more easily, so it is best to keep the hooves dry, using a hoof sealer if necessary.

CONTRACTED HEELS

Contraction of one or both heels of a hoof can be caused by LT-LH configuration, lack of use of the foot (such as when the limb is injured and nonweight-bearing for a period of time or when the horse's exercise is restricted) or physical restriction of the hoof by horseshoe nails, clips, bandaging or cast.

Identification of contracted heels can be made by the following method: the width of the heels ¼ inch from the buttresses should equal or exceed the width of the trimmed hoof 1 inch back from the toe. If the heel measurement is less than the toe measurement, the

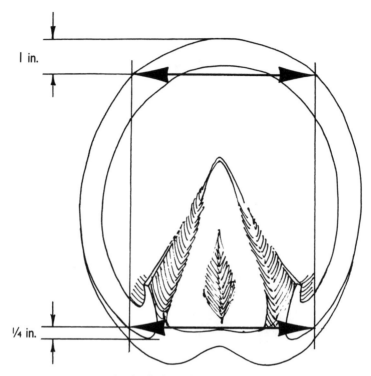

One method of identifying contracted heels

heels are said to be contracted. However, some horses have a con-
genital or adapted hoof shape that fits the definition of contracted
heels, but the hoof is balanced by other criteria and the animal is
sound. In these cases, it is not advisable to try to spread the heels.

As a hoof deviates toward LT-LH, the hoof elongates from toe to
heel and the heels generally get closer together. When the horse's
weight rotates over the long toe in a prolonged breakover, the heels of
the hoof are drawn inward. Balancing the hoof and shoeing with a
squared-toe shoe that provides adequate heel support allows such a
hoof to function more normally and encourages the heels to spread.

When a horse lacks exercise, the blood flow in the foot is decreased,
causing a drop in the moisture content of the hoof capsule. In the idle
horse, the lack of pressure pushing outward from the descending
weight of the horse during movement coupled with an increased
inward-curling force from the drying outer hoof wall causes the hoof
capsule to contract at the heels. This contraction can compress the sensitive inner structures of the hoof resulting in lameness or soreness.

The treatment is to increase the exercise level of the horse and retard the evaporation of internal moisture by application of a hoof sealer (see Resource Guide in the Appendix). In some instances a shoe with slippered heels may be applied until the hoof regains its shape. The heel portion of the bearing surface of this shoe is sloped outward to physically spread the hoof as the horse's weight descends. If the horse cannot be exercised, the moisture content of the hoof might need to be increased by wet bandages or by placing the horse in a stall with damp sand or sawdust. Other, more dramatic mechanical devices have been used to physically spread the heels of a contracted hoof, but these are futile without removing the cause of contraction.

When the hoof must be in a cast or restrictive shoe for a long period to treat an injury, the heels usually will contract. A similar contraction may result from consistently nailing on shoes with the nails too far back toward the heels. The last two nail holes on many factory-made shoes are behind the widest part of the hoof. These last two nails should usually be omitted unless specifically used to restrict the expansion of a bilaterally flared hoof. In most cases, the hoof will return to normal when the restriction is removed, the hoof is balanced and the horse resumes regular exercise.

LONG TOE–LOW HEEL (LT-LH) AND UNDERRUN HEELS

When proper DP hoof balance is not maintained by trimming and/or shoeing, the hoof attains an abnormal LT-LH configuration which can result in excess flexor tendon stress and cause heel soreness, cracks, contracted heels and development of the navicular syndrome.

The LT-LH configuration can occur in several ways: a horse with poor-quality hoof horn is left barefoot; the hooves are not trimmed regularly and grow a long toe; the horse receives poor trimming and shoeing; the horse is overdue for shoeing.

If the heel is trimmed too short and the toe is left too long and a shoe is placed on the hoof, the hoof angle is fixed at the outset at a too-low angle and it becomes worse as the hoof grows. Even with a properly balanced hoof, if the shoe is left on too long, the heels will expand over the shoe and the horn at the heels will be crushed, while the toe grows longer and is prevented from wear by the shoe.

The LT-LH configuration places excess stress on the flexor tendons and navicular region and can cause underrun heels, an often irreversible condition where the angle of the hoof horn at the heels is lower than the toe angle by 5 degrees or more.

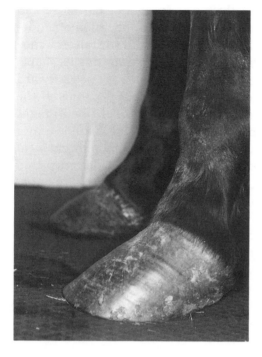

Way overdue for a trim

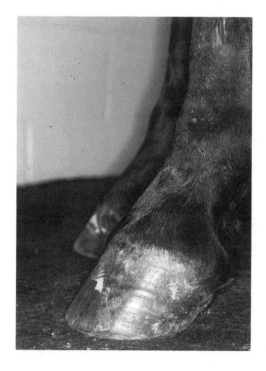

Same horse after a trim

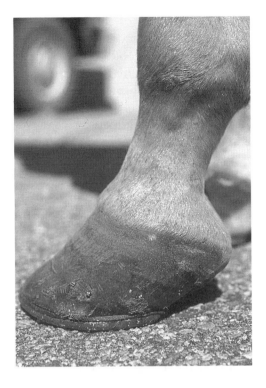

Way overdue for proper shoeing

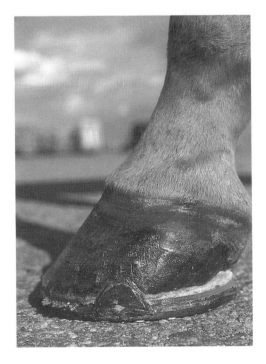

Same horse after shoeing with egg bar and full pad

In trimming a hoof with *low* heels, the toe of the hoof wall is trimmed as short as is practical, tapering off toward the quarters. The heels are taken down only enough to get a good bearing surface of healthy horn, and this can often be accomplished more precisely with the rasp alone, minimizing the risk of trimming them too much (see figure on page 43).

However, *underrun* heels should often be trimmed short so the support for the hoof is more rearward. Leaving underrun heels long in an attempt to align the hoof-pastern axis only forces the heels to grow farther forward underneath the limb and creates an open invitation for lost shoes. After trimming the heels very short, the hoof-pastern axis can be aligned by elevating the heels with wedge-heel shoes or wedge pads (degree pads). An alternative is to rebuild the heels to a normal length and angle with a prosthetic hoof material (see Resource Guide in the Appendix). The hoof can then be shod in a normal manner.

SYMPTOMS ASSOCIATED WITH NAVICULAR SYNDROME

Numbers 1 through 4 are the most classic symptoms

1. A history of progressive, chronic forelimb lameness involving one or both limbs.
2. A stiff, shuffling gait with a short, choppy stride.
3. Sensitivity to hoof testers when the central third of the frog is compressed.
4. A positive response to nerve "blocking" (low palmar digital nerve block).
5. Pointing of the most severely affected forelimb or alternate pointing.
6. Low, underrun heels.
7. Broken back hoof/pastern axis.
8. One forefoot smaller and more upright.
9. Contracted heels in one or both feet.
10. Toe-first landing when walking or trotting.
11. Occasional stumbling.
12. When circling, lameness of the inside foot more exaggerated and head carried to outside of circle.
13. A marked lameness after a sharp turn.
14. A pain response and/or increase in lameness in response to the interphalangeal flexion test.

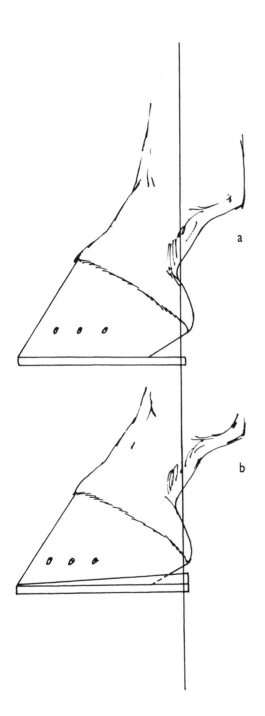

Although a and b provide
adequate support, b will more
likely correct underrun heels
and result in fewer lost shoes.

NAVICULAR SYNDROME

Navicular syndrome is a chronic forelimb lameness involving the navicular bone and associated structures. Signs of navicular syndrome are outlined on page 170. Not all lamenesses associated with the heel area of the hoof, however, should be attributed to navicular syndrome. Factors thought to predispose a horse to navicular problems include poor conformation, improper or irregular shoeing and stress to the navicular region. A common error that can lead to navicular syndrome is associated with the false economy of stretching the intervals between shoeings. As a hoof grows past its optimum reset time, the toe gets too long and the heel too low, resulting in a broken back axis. Increased pressure between the deep flexor tendon and the navicular bone may cause the heel pain associated with navicular syndrome (see figure on page 43).

The egg bar shoe (Chapter 6) has proven of great value in the treatment of the navicular syndrome. It is a noninvasive, inexpensive treatment with virtually no negative side effects or risks. In addition, the egg bar shoe has positive effects on hoof conformation.

Some horses show dramatic clinical improvement soon after egg bar shoes are applied, as if their call for support was answered. However, some underrun hooves have gone past a critical horn tubule

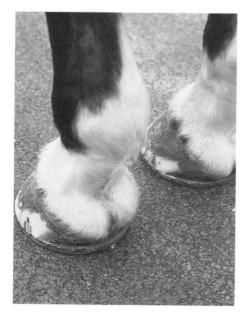

Egg bar shoes

angle and have reached the point of no return. Even though these hooves will not likely show a reversal of the underrun heel condition, the horse may be usable and comfortable working in egg bar shoes or full support shoes for many years.

Full pads are often prescribed for horses that have navicular syndrome. Hooves with wide open, low heels are sometimes believed to have incurred navicular disease or heel soreness from the direct concussion to the frog and heel area. Full pads used to *protect* this area can actually *transmit* the concussion to the navicular region. A straight pad or full support shoe might be more effective in providing protection for this type of navicular problem (Chapter 6).

WRY HOOF

A wry hoof is a deformation that is usually, but not always, associated with sheared heels. The entire hoof wall when viewed from the front appears to sweep off to one side. In the case of a hoof that is wry to the inside, the medial wall will flare inward and the outer wall will curl in underneath the hoof. A wry hoof is caused primarily by ML imbalance. This imbalance can be the result of improper trimming; from pain in the limb, which causes the horse to land more heavily on one side of the hoof, or from the way in which the hoof is worn as the horse turns in a habitual way in a stall or pen.

To return a wry hoof to a normal configuration, the flare is dressed off and the hoof is shod with a bar shoe that is centered beneath the limb. This means that the shoe will extend beyond the turned-under hoof wall by as much as ¼ to ⅜ inch, and will be shod very close to the wall on the flared side.

The remaining hooves should be checked closely for balance, because abnormalities affecting the shape of one hoof will often affect the other hooves, usually the diagonal limb.

SHEARED HEELS

ML imbalance (Chapter 5) can lead to sheared heels and cracks. On a straight limb, lines from the coronet to the ground on the medial and lateral sides of the hoof will be the same length, and the coronet will form a smooth line around the top of the hoof. The hoof will strike the ground flat (both sides simultaneously) at a walk.

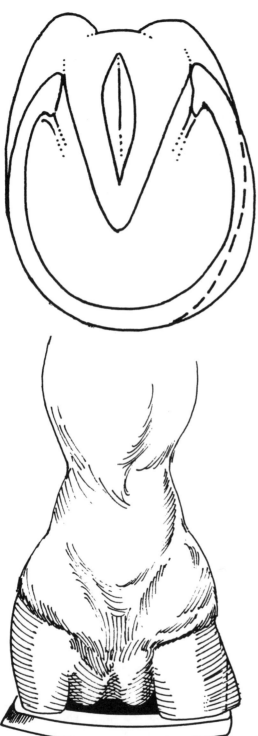

Removing a flare

Shoeing the wry hoof

When one side of the hoof becomes too short through wear or trimming, uneven stress is placed on the entire hoof structure. When a disproportionate amount of weight is borne by one side of the hoof, the entire side of the hoof wall can be dislocated upward, actually shearing the heels between the bulbs. Grasping a heel of a sheared hoof in each hand, one can often move the heels independently. Some horse's hoof structure adapts to this sheared configuration over many years, making a return to normal impossible, and in some cases undesirable. If imbalanced during the formative years, a hoof may be permanently fixed into that abnormal balance, which then becomes "normal" for that horse. A recent development of sheared heels, often causing soreness and lameness, can usually be remedied by therapeutic shoeing methods.

If a small area of the hoof wall is allowed to be too long (such as when the shoe does not fit flat on the hoof) or if a small area of the hoof is growing faster, focal pressure is directed up the hoof wall, which can cause a section of the coronet to be displaced upward. A coronet displacement often goes undetected and can be the cause of subtle lameness.

The treatment for sheared heels is to allow the displaced hoof wall to drop down to its original position. The hoof is trimmed in balance as if it were not sheared, and a bar shoe is fit to the hoof. Before the bar shoe is applied, the ground surface of the displaced heel is further trimmed ("floated") so that it will not bear on the shoe. There should be a gap of ¼ to ½ inch between the shoe and the hoof, tapering to meet at midquarter. Some hooves will remodel in one or two shoeings. Other longstanding cases may never return to normal.

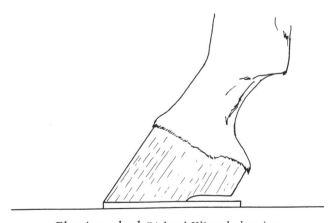

Floating a heel. Richard Klimesh drawing

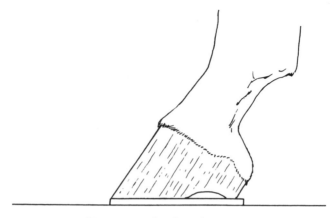

Treating a displaced coronet.
Richard Klimesh drawing

The treatment for a displaced coronet is similar to that for sheared heels. Below the site of the displacement (following the horn tubules to the ground surface) the hoof wall is sculpted out to parallel the bulge at the coronet. This allows the displaced area of the hoof wall to descend to the shoe and the coronet to assume its normal position.

This re-forming of the hoof is often facilitated (after trimming in the above manner) by leaving the shoes off of the affected hooves and keeping the horse in a stall with a base of damp sand or a deep layer of dampened course sawdust for several days. The hoof will re-form (and de-form) more readily with a greater moisture content, and this footing will support the entire ground surface of the hoof, allowing the hoof wall to settle down to a normal level. The hooves might also be encouraged in this remodeling by wrapping them with moist bandages and by periodically rasping the ground surface of the hoof at the site of displacement as it settles.

CRACKS

Cracks are separations or breaks in the hoof wall. Vertical cracks between the tubules that comprise the hoof horn are referred to by their location, such as toe cracks, quarter cracks and heel cracks. Cracks that originate at the coronet are called sand cracks, while those that start at the ground surface are called grass cracks.

A horizontal crack in the hoof wall is called a blow-out. Blow-outs are caused either by an injury to the coronary band or by a blow to

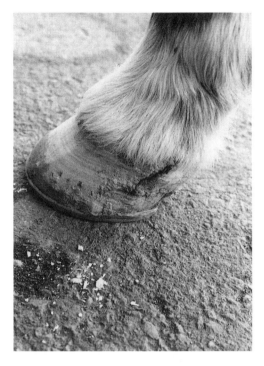

Quarter crack

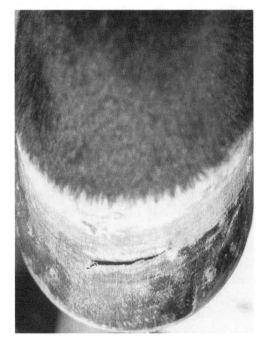

Blow-out crack

the hoof wall. A blow-out usually will not result in lameness and many times will go unnoticed until the farrier spots it. Once they occur, these cracks seldom increase in size horizontally and usually require no treatment. However, because the hoof is weaker at this site, a blow-out can set the stage for a vertical crack if the hoof is weakened by excess moisture or is not in ML balance.

Cracks do not "heal" back together. The hoof wall must be replaced primarily by new growth from the coronary band, just as a damaged fingernail must grow out. This will take from nine to twelve months. For optimum hoof growth, it is essential that the ration contains nutrients necessary for healthy hoof horn (Chapter 14); (see Resource Guide in the Appendix).

Sand cracks can result from an injury to the coronet or from an infection in the foot that breaks out at the coronet. Sometimes a horse will bump the coronet when loading or unloading from a trailer, or the horse might strike his coronet during fast work or an uncoordinated movement.

A wet environment containing sand or gravel can soften a horse's hooves and allow particles to be forced up into the white line. If infection results, it can travel upward through the laminae and break out at the coronet, possibly causing a crack to form. Cracks often appear at the site of a displaced coronet.

The first step in dealing with sand cracks is to determine the cause and remove it. This, accompanied by a good shoeing, may be all that is necessary to stabilize the hoof, as it replaces the damaged horn. Severe cracks can be held immobile by a variety of methods until the hoof grows out. These have included nailing or screwing across the crack, drilling holes on either side and lacing the crack up like a boot, fastening a metal plate across the crack, and patching the crack together with plastic, fiberglass or other types of materials.

Today the farrier and veterinarian can choose from several high-tech acrylic materials developed specifically to bond to the hoof wall. Some of these materials mimic the consistency of the hoof wall so that once applied they can be nailed into, trimmed and rasped along with the hoof wall as it grows down. The prosthetic materials can be used to completely fill the crack or to form a patch across the crack. (See Resource Guide in the Appendix.)

Before the crack can be stabilized, it must be thoroughly cleansed of dirt, loose hoof horn and bacteria. If there is any evidence of moist tissue, the crack must be treated by a veterinarian until it is completely dry. Applying any type of patching material over a moist crack would seal in bacteria, providing the perfect environment for an infection to develop or escalate.

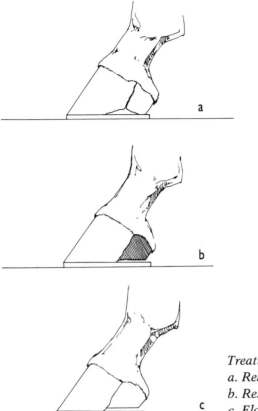

Treating a crack
a. Relieving
b. Resecting
c. Floating

Chronic or very severe cracks toward the heel of the hoof are some-times dealt with by removing the section of the hoof wall behind the crack. The hoof is then supported by a full support shoe (Chapter 6) until new hoof grows down. A similar but less involved approach is to apply a full support shoe and "float" the portion of the hoof behind the crack. Floating means to trim that portion of the hoof about ¼ inch shorter so it will not contact the shoe. By eliminating weight-bearing behind the crack, movement of the two halves of the crack is minimized, and the hoof will often grow down intact. A horse that is very active or in work, however, will likely need to have the crack more securely stabilized.

Grass cracks most often appear in unshod hooves that have been allowed to grow too long. Often all that is needed to control these cracks is a good trimming. More severe cracks may require shoes for several months until new hoof tissue can grow down and replace the

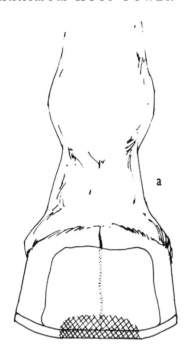

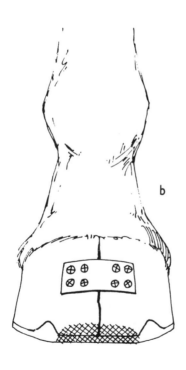

Stabilizing a Crack
a. Acrylic patch
b. Screwed-on plate

cracked horn. To help toe cracks grow out, the hoof angle must be kept up where it belongs and a square-toed shoe applied to minimize the prying effect of breakover.

Surface cracks are tiny fissures that cover varying portions of the hoof wall. They are most often caused by a change in hoof moisture, such as when a horse on wet pasture is put in a stall with dry bedding or when a horse that has been standing in mud then stands in the sun. Surface cracks are remedied by stabilizing the horse's moisture balance, minimizing his exposure to wetness and using a hoof sealer. Thick hoof dressings may fill the cracks and improve the exterior appearance of a hoof, but a hoof sealer is more beneficial to long-term hoof health (see Resource Guide in the Appendix).

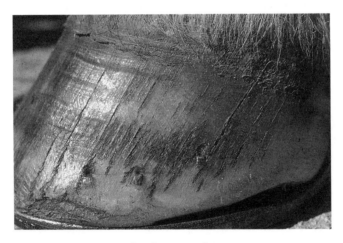

Surface cracks

BRUISES, CORNS AND ABSCESSES

When the hoof is trimmed, the outer wall should be long enough so it, not the sole, is the primary weight-bearing structure. Pressure on the perimeter of the sole inside the white line can cause pain and can compress the blood vessels beneath the sole. If the wall is trimmed too short, if the sole is very flat or if a barefoot horse has worn its hooves so short that the soles are flat or protruding below the hoof wall, the sole will likely be bruised (see photograph on page 19). Horses in muddy pens, shod or not, will often bruise their soles when the temperature drops and the lumpy mud freezes hard.

Normally the healthy sole has a concave shape, like a shallow bowl, and is about ¼ inch thick on a saddle horse. A properly trimmed sole will only "give," or have springiness, under *very heavy* thumb pressure. If the sole gives to *moderate* pressure, it may be too short to adequately protect the inner structures from bruising, especially on rocky or frozen ground. A thin-soled horse may lack confidence of movement and be "off." Bruising may develop into an abscess that can cause varying degrees of lameness. The abscess can even affect the coffin bone, causing a life-threatening situation. If a thin sole is the result of recent trimming, the horse, even when shod, may be uncomfortable when walked over gravel or rough ground. In a week or so, the sole will thicken enough for the horse to be comfortable.

Corns are bruises or abscesses that occur inside the buttress where the hoof wall curves to join the bars. This site is actually referred to as "the seat of corn." Corns are usually caused by pressure from a horseshoe or from a stone wedged between the shoe and the hoof. When the hoof is trimmed, the seat of corn should be pared below the level of the hoof wall to prevent contact with the shoe. If the shoe is left on too long and the hoof overgrows the shoe, the heels often collapse and pressure is put on the seat of corn, resulting in a bruise or abscess. A corn can cause varying degrees of lameness. Trimming to remove pressure on the corn may be all that is required. If the corn is infected, it is treated as an abscess.

Full pads are often used to protect a bruised sole while it heals, but, if a pad is applied over a sole bruise that is on the verge of abscess, it will tend to fester the abscess quickly. The horse may exhibit great pain a day or so after the pad has been applied, necessitating the removal of the pad. Once the abscess has been treated by a veterinarian and has dried out, a pad can be reapplied, if needed.

HOT NAIL

A horseshoe nail driven into the hoof wall that puts pressure on the sensitive inner structures without actually piercing them is referred to as a close nail. A close nail may cause the horse immediate discomfort or may go unnoticed for many days or until the horse is put into work. Usually the offending nail can be located by the use of a hoof tester or by judicious tapping with a hammer at the location of

Nail Path

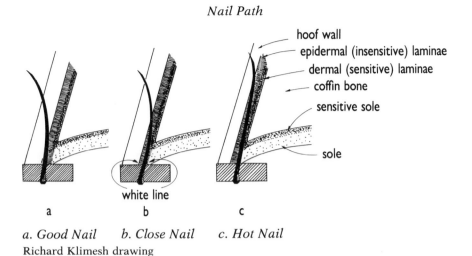

a. *Good Nail*   b. *Close Nail*   c. *Hot Nail*
Richard Klimesh drawing

each nail. Removal of the close nail will often return the horse to soundness, since the sensitive structures have not been invaded.

A nail that is driven *into* the sensitive structures of the hoof is called a hot nail. A hot nail will usually cause the horse to exhibit immediate pain unless the horse is under sedation. If the animal is normally fractious when being shod, the response to a hot nail may go unnoticed. Upon removing a hot nail, blood will likely be seen in the nail hole and on the nail itself. The hole should be flushed with an antiseptic such as betadine and plugged to prevent contamination. A nail should not be placed in the hole. The horse should be current on its tetanus vaccination and should be observed for several days for continuing or developing lameness.

If an abscess develops, a veterinarian should be contacted. Usually the shoe is removed and the hoof is soaked in hot water—Epsom salts solution twice daily for two to three days. When the veterinarian determines that the infection has cleared, the shoe can be replaced.

THRUSH

Thrush is caused by an anaerobic bacteria that thrives in the warm, dark recesses of the hoof. The bacteria's foul-smelling black exudate is most commonly found in the clefts of the frog and if left untreated can invade sensitive tissues, especially deep in the central cleft, and cause lameness. Thrush will also inhabit separations and cracks in the hoof wall, especially if the horse is in a moist environment. Cleanliness is the best prevention and the first step of any treatment program. "Sugardine" is very effective for treating thrush: a thin paste is made from white sugar and betadine scrub and spread on the cleaned areas daily until the problem is resolved. Commercial preparations for treating thrush are available and are effective in varying degrees. Severe cases of thrush can be treated with the CVP Gasket Pad (Chapter 6).

WHITE LINE DISEASE

When an area of separation occurs in the hoof wall, it provides a moist dark environment, ideal for the growth of horn-digesting organisms. Soil and manure may be forced up into the interlaminar space as the white line deteriorates. If left unchecked, this situation can progress to white line disease and result in lameness and much expense.

White line disease, sometimes called seedy toe, is due to invasion of the inner horn by bacteria, fungus, and/or yeast, which results in varying degrees of damage to the structural integrity of the hoof. There seems to be a greater occurrence of the condition in hot, humid climates.

The area of an affected hoof is characteristically filled with a white cheesy material and air pockets that are often packed with debris. The disease starts at ground level and if not controlled can work its way up to the coronary band.

An affected horse may show symptoms similar to those of laminitis: lameness, heat, sole tending to be flat, slow horn growth, tenderness when nailing and pain over the sole when hoof testers are applied. There may be areas of the hoof wall that when tapped give a hollow sound. Depending on the extent of the damage, lameness can result from mechanical loss of horn support. In severe cases, the destruction of the laminae may cause a rotation of the coffin bone.

Any separation in the white line should be considered a seed for seedy toe. A separation is often found between the heel and the quarter in the white line. The cavity may be ¼ inch deep or extend halfway up the hoof wall. The space is usually filled with a white chalky substance or thrush's foul smelling, tarlike residue. These heel caves can be treated by digging out as much of the decomposed horn as possible and packing the hole using the CVP method (Chapter 6). If the hole is very deep, the treatment materials may need to be layered. A shoe is applied to protect the packing and to prevent further contamination. The horse should be kept in a dry environment and the shoes reset regularly, at which time the packing is replaced. The hoof deterioration will usually be prevented from spreading with this treatment, and the hoof will grow down solid. If the area of separation is very large or extends for a distance along the white line, the above treatment is used in conjunction with the application of a CVP Gasket Pad. Treatment of severe cases of white line disease may involve a partial resection of the undermined hoof wall by a vet.

BOWED TENDON

An inflammation of the flexor tendon (usually the superficial flexor tendon of the front limb) is called a bowed tendon. Flexor tendon strain is the main cause of bowed tendon. The strain can be brought about by poor hoof and limb conformation (long, weak pasterns), poor or irregular shoeing (lack of adequate support), muscle fatigue, heavy footing, a misstep and work at speed.

Even if a hoof is trimmed to a proper hoof angle, if the shoe that is applied is too short and does not provide adequate tendon support, problems may result (see figure on page 52). And as a hoof grows longer, the attached shoe migrates forward on the hoof so the heels of the shoe end up farther forward than they started. If the shoe is fit flush with the heels at the start, in six weeks the shoe will not even cover the hoof at the heels, let alone support it. If a horse is in heavy work, a good form of insurance against bowed tendons would be extended heels or egg bar shoes.

ARTHRITIS

Arthritis is a general term for joint inflammation. It describes a range of conditions affecting any joint in the body. It is usually chronic but has acute signs. There are various names for arthritis in specific joints, such as

jack spavin or bone spavin = hock arthritis
osselets = fetlock arthritis
ringbone = pastern and/or coffin joint arthritis

Degenerative joint disease (DJD), also called osteoarthritis, refers to a group of disorders that end with deterioration of articular cartilage and changes in the bone and soft tissues of the joint.

The chain of events leading to arthritis can be complex and inter-related. The initial cause may be hard use, a fall, a blow to the joint, poor conformation, inadequate conditioning or inadequate farrier care. Affected joints show a decreased range of motion. Treatment aims at relieving pain and preventing further damage. In some cases, farrier adjustments are necessary to remove the primary cause of arthritic pain. Balancing the hoof and removing traction devices are the most common adjustments. Using a plain or wide-web shoe will allow the horse to slide as it lands. Using a shock-absorbing pad may give the horse some relief. Horses with bone spavin may get relief from wedge heels or wedge pads with a squared or rocker toe shoe.

COFFIN BONE FRACTURE

Horses turning at speed (barrel racing, roping, jumping) sometimes fracture a coffin bone. Depending on the location and severity of the fracture, it is possible that treatment can restore the horse to its previous level of performance. The Klimesh Contiguous Clip Shoe may be helpful in this regard (Chapter 6). The shoe effectively im-mobilizes the hoof capsule and the coffin bone inside. Depending on the configuration of the hoof and the management of the horse's en-vironment, it may be necessary to use a full pad or a metal plate to prevent trauma to the coffin bone through the bottom of the hoof. The shoe will need to be reset or replaced at four- to six-week intervals for six months or a year. When lameness is no longer evident and the X rays show satisfactory healing, the hoof can be shod with a bar shoe and two side clips to stabilize the hoof and prevent refracture.

LAMINITIS

Laminitis is an acute inflammation of the sensitive laminae in the hoof, which can be caused by a wide variety of factors including overeating of grain or pasture, trauma and foaling complications. The chronic form of the condition is often referred to as founder. It is likely that a number of horses experience mild laminitis and recover without it ever being recognized. Other horses that experience mild laminitis may or may not be diagnosed as such by the veterinarian and may recover and return to normal work with or without (or in spite of) treatment.

Horses that suffer significant hoof damage from laminitis, resulting in weeks or months of unsoundness, are unlikely to ever return to their previous level of performance. Some of these horses can become sound enough for light turnout. However, mares so affected may not be able to bear the additional weight of a pregnancy without refoundering.

Successful laminitis treatment involves a cooperative effort from the horse owner, veterinarian and farrier. Although an experienced veterinarian and farrier can set the stage for a horse's recovery, the owner's long-term commitment to the treatment program is of paramount importance. Dealing with laminitis can require emotional strength and a considerable investment of time and money. Besides initial emergency care, a horse suffering from severe laminitis will need frequent farrier attention and periodic veterinary care for a year or more. Most cases will require daily treatment, specialized management and close supervision for life. Some horses, in spite of conscientious treatment and care, will fail to improve and may worsen. Since laminitis is the second leading cause (next to colic) of equine death, prevention is essential. Monitor your horse's weight closely, be certain your horse cannot get into the feed room and carefully select and monitor the horses you turn out on pasture. For more information, see the Recommended Reading list in the Appendix.

CLUB FOOT

A DP imbalance at the other end of the scale from LT-LH is the club foot, which is essentially a short toe–long heel. This type of imbalance often affects a hoof that has been nonweight-bearing for a period of time, because of an injury, for example. In this case the club foot is usually temporary in nature and can be coached back to a normal shape by judicious trimming and proper exercise.

Another type of mild club foot is caused by excessive wear of the bare toe from pawing, toe dragging or poor-quality hoof wall. This type of club foot can often be controlled by application of a half shoe, also called a tip shoe. Usually made from the toe portion of a light shoe like a training plate, the half shoe protects the toe of the hoof and leaves the heels bare to wear off in a normal fashion. The ends of the half shoe are tapered and/or set into the hoof so there is not an abrupt step where the shoe makes the transition to the quarters of the hoof. If the toe of the hoof is worn back, the toe of the half shoe can be extended out to the normal point of breakover. A side benefit of the half shoe is that it cannot be stepped off!

A more serious type of club foot is caused by a contraction of the flexor muscle–tendon unit that attaches to the coffin bone (see figure on page 13). This club foot may occur in one or both feet. It most commonly affects the fronts. The reasons for this contracture are not clearly understood, but as the tendon tightens, it pulls the heels of the hoof off the ground and they tend to grow very long. The horse's weight is shifted onto the toe, which causes excessive wear and a dishing of the toe.

Trying to forcibly lower the heels of this type of club foot is rarely a good idea. In most cases, such an approach will make the club foot worse. It is better to support the heels by an elevated shoe or a shoe in conjunction with a wedge pad. If, when the horse is standing squarely, there is ¼ inch of space between the heels of the club foot and the ground, the amount of elevation should be ½ inch or more. This procedure allows the heels to bear weight, takes some weight off the toe, and lessens the constant strain on the deep flexor muscle–tendon unit. Sometimes this will break the contraction cycle, allowing the muscle to relax enough so the hoof can be gradually lowered down over a period of weeks to a more normal angle. In other cases, the horse may never be able to have its heels lowered but may be comfortable and even usable with the elevated heels.

Foals with mild to moderate club feet, if diagnosed and treated early, have a fair chance to perform unencumbered as adults. Advances in glue-on shoe technology allow corrective shoes to be applied to foals at a few weeks of age. However, it is difficult to predict which foals will respond to treatment. Yearlings that have had extensive corrective trimming and shoeing to correct club feet may appear normal, but radiographs may show malformations of the coffin bone. Changes in the coffin bone usually indicate a poor chance for the young horse to perform as athletes.

MISMATCHED FEET

Mismatched feet, or high-low syndrome, usually affects the front feet. One hoof tends toward LT-LH and the other tends to be clubby. Some farriers report that over half of the horses they shoe have mismatched feet to some degree.

One approach to dealing with the high-low syndrome is to lower the heels of the steep hoof and elevate the heels of the low hoof so hoof angles match. Where the initial difference between the feet is slight (less than 5 degrees), this method usually works fine and will not affect the horse's performance.

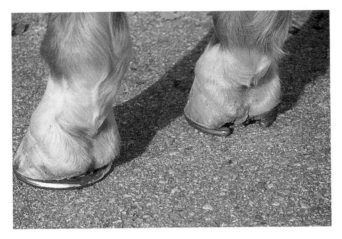

Mismatched limbs often require different support.

However, if the difference in toe angles is 5 degrees or greater, it is usually better not to force the hooves to be the same angle. Mismatched feet on a sound horse are more "balanced" than matching feet on a lame horse. This is why some farriers shun the use of a hoof gauge as a trimming guide. They feel that it is better to align the hoof and pastern of each foot visually and to evaluate the horse's movement when determining how to trim.

To attain dynamic balance and an even stride, it may be necessary to shoe a horse with two different shoes on the fronts. For example, a horse might wear a squared-toe egg bar on the low hoof and a thicker, full-toed plain shoe on the steep hoof. The egg bar will provide support for the low heels and the squared toe will help speed breakover. The thicker shoe on the steep hoof will make up for the extra weight of the egg bar on the low hoof. The lower hoof seems to have more natural "action" anyway, and the steep hoof may need an even heavier shoe to balance the movement. This symmetry of limb movement is more important for horses that are being judged in the ring on the correctness of their gaits. With most horses, however, it is sufficient to concentrate on shoeing to provide necessary support.

When trimming mismatched feet, it is easy to trim the steep hoof too short. That's why it is best to trim the low hoof first and then the steep hoof only enough to match the toe lengths. One method of evaluating relative toe lengths is to stand the horse on a flat, level surface and view the knees from the front. The bumps on the insides of the knees should usually be the same level. If necessary, a rim pad or wedge pad can be used to elevate the low hoof.

Teamwork

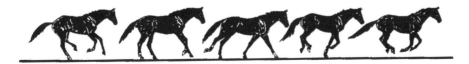

Training a Horse for Shoeing

If you want your farrier to do his best work and look forward to coming back to your barn, train your horses to be cooperative and relaxed for shoeing. It is not in your farrier's job description to train your horse. And it is unfair for you to expect him to take the time and to risk injury by handling an untrained horse. If you raise young horses, begin early with their training. A horse should be able to do all of the following before a farrier is asked to work on him:

• Stand tied without pulling back.
• Stand still while tied, unless asked to move.
• Stand tied without pawing.
• Pick up all four feet cooperatively.
• Stand in balance when any leg is held for two minutes without moving, leaning, trying to pull his leg away, fidgeting or nibbling.
• Move sideways to the left and right on cue one step at a time while tied.
• Back up and step forward on cue one step at a time while tied.
• Allow all four legs to be brought backward.
• Allow all four legs to be brought forward on a hoof stand or knee for at least thirty seconds.

Many foals require corrective rasping of their hooves at two months of age or earlier. To prepare the foal for the farrier's first visit, hold a regular series of hoof-handling lessons. They should begin the first day of the foal's life, when you accustom the foal to being caught and having its body and legs handled. When the foal is a week old,

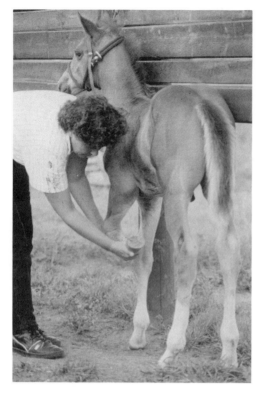

Training the suckling foal

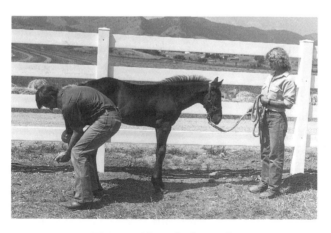

*This suckling foal stands
quietly for the farrier.*

you should be able to pick up a leg and hold it, with a competent handler holding the foal with a halter alongside the stall wall or a sturdy fence. (It is best to have the mare tied nearby.) At first just pick the legs up briefly, but increase the amount of time to at least thirty seconds per leg. (An older horse will be expected to hold a leg up for two to three minutes.) This will condition the foal to stand still long enough for the farrier to trim his hooves. When you can hold the leg without struggle, gently bend the hoof from side to side and from front to back. This accustoms the foal to the movements the farrier will make during trimming.

A properly conditioned foal will likely retain his good manners throughout his life, but leg-handling lessons should be reviewed to reinforce manners and to decrease the chance of injury should the horse get caught in rope or wire. All yearlings and two-year-olds should receive a formal series of conditioning and restraint lessons by a competent, experienced trainer. The procedure is outlined in detail in *The Formative Years* (see Recommended Reading in the Appendix).

So that a horse of any age is comfortable having his legs handled and the lessons proceed safely, follow these guidelines:

1. Work in close to the horse's body. This helps restrain the horse, gives a horse an added measure of confidence and is safer for the handler.

2. Minimize the amount of sideways pull you exert on the horse's leg. Try to lift the leg in the plane in which it normally moves, that is, underneath the horse's body. With a tiny foal, this may require you to crouch down to the foal's level.

3. Never let your horse decide when it is time to put his foot down. *You* choose the moment. It should be when the horse is standing quietly, not struggling. Then place the hoof decisively on the ground (don't let it just drop).

4. When you are picking up a left leg, push the horse's weight over to the horse's right shoulder or hip with your shoulder or elbow.

5. Don't try to pick up a hoof by force. Rather, take advantage of the horse's inborn withdrawal reflex. When a wild horse's leg is touched by a branch or a buzzing fly, the horse's automatic reaction is to pick up his leg, often very quickly and high. Your domestic horse will still exhibit this reflex, especially if you touch it in a strategic area. But because you will also want to be able to groom, bandage and clip your horse's legs *without* him picking them up, you must teach him to differentiate between your command to pick up a foot and the one that tells him to keep his feet on the ground.

To teach him to pick his foot up, give the voice command "Foot," and at the same time pinch the tendon area above the fetlock. The

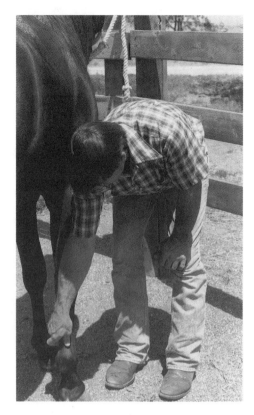

Pinching the tendon

pinching will cause your horse to pick up his foot. Be ready to catch his hoof or he will put it back down as part of the reflex cycle. With time you can teach your horse to respond to the voice command alone.

6. Once you have grasped the hoof, hold it in a natural position without pulling the leg outward or overflexing the joints. If the process is made comfortable for a horse, especially for a foal, he will be less likely to struggle. If a horse does try to pull his leg away from you, you will have a better chance of hanging on if you tip the toe up so the fetlock and pastern are hyperflexed. This tends to block nerve transmissions and reflexes. With very "thin-skinned" sensitive horses, it sometimes is better to hold onto the hoof rather than the leg for the first few lessons.

7. Use generous body-to-body contact to assure the horse that your control is not tenuous. However, do not allow or encourage your horse to lean on you. Although it may not be difficult to support part of the body weight of a 100-pound foal, it won't take long before that foal is a 1,200-pound animal. If he has learned that leaning is okay, he will likely retain the habit for life.

8. When bringing the hind leg of a young or short horse backward, take care not to raise the leg too high (to accommodate the height of your "lap"), as this may cause the horse discomfort in the joints, especially the stifle. Many times the reason a horse struggles is because his joints are being stressed due to improper leg lifting. If you are lifting the hind leg of a young or small horse in a conscientious fashion and the horse struggles because of impatience or poor temper, you can sometimes retain a hold on him by using a "hock lock." Drape your arm nearest the horse over his hock. With your other hand, tip the toe of the hoof up. This gives you a leverage advantage in the event the young horse tries to pull away. The competency of the person on the lead rope will have a big effect on how a horse of any age behaves while having his legs handled.

HORSE BEHAVIOR DURING SHOEING

A knowledgeable farrier usually doesn't mind a curious young horse briefly inspecting him and his tools with polite sniffing. However, dishonest nibbling when the farrier's back is to the horse (which is 90% of the time) is unacceptable. To prevent such a habit from forming, as you train your horse, use "farrier positions" (such as drawing a front leg forward on your knee as if a hoof stand) to "bait" and test your horse. If your horse sees this as an opportunity to nibble, either discipline him using a bop on the nose with the back of your upper arm or a tug on his lead rope or chain, or have an assistant reprimand the horse.

If a horse is not sufficiently confident when separated from other horses, he may desperately attempt to retain communication with or physical proximity to his buddies. The chronic case is referred to as herd bound or barn sour: the insecure horse links comfort, companionship and food with the barn, a particular stall or with certain horses. What your farrier has to deal with is a horse that screams, paws, swerves sideways, defecates repeatedly and in general pays more attention to where his buddies are than to the farrier working on him. This is very unsafe (and nerve-racking) for your farrier. What may seem to be a "normal" insecurity in a young or inexperienced horse may evolve into a long-standing and dangerous habit.

Ideally, a horse should be "weaned" from its herdmates just as it was from its mother. This should be approached as a systematic training project, however, not begun the morning of your farrier's visit. If young horses are routinely kept in separate pens or stalls or

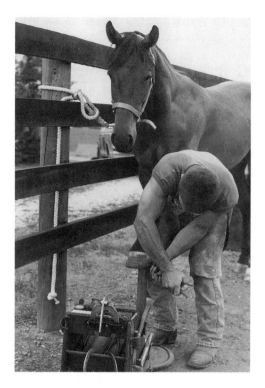

This yearling's first shoeing occurs without nibbling or pulling the hoof off the stand.

periodically tied alone to a hitching post for several hours at a time, they soon accept separation and begin developing a healthy self-confidence.

One of the underlying obstacles in getting any horse to stand still is the fact that horses are born wanderers. When the nomadic tendency is thwarted by excessive confinement or improperly applied restraint and embellished by excessive feed and inadequate exercise, vices such as pawing, weaving and pacing can result. Regular exercise is essential for the horse's physical and mental well-being. A fresh horse, even if well trained, might fidget when asked to stand still for shoeing. A very high-strung horse that has inadequate exercise is overreactive, often nervous and generally unsafe.

An exhausted horse is not the answer either. Such a horse will probably be tuned out and unresponsive, and will likely lean on the farrier. Some horses learn these lazy habits because a timid owner doesn't know how to encourage the horse to cooperate. Most horses can be taught in a simple and nonaggressive way to pick up their feet and hold them up without leaning.

Although most horses defecate unabashedly while being shod, few will urinate, especially if the shoeing area is a hard floor that splatters back. If a normally cooperative horse becomes extremely rest-less, give him the opportunity to relieve himself in a bedded stall.

The timing of a farrier appointment can affect a horse's behavior. If a particular horse's time to be shod comes just as his exercise buddies are being turned out, he may be thinking of running more than standing still. Although a horse should be expected to cooperate with fair demands any time, anywhere, it might make your farrier's job less pleasant if he has to shoe your horse when feed buckets are banging, stall doors are sliding open and closed, traffic in the aisle is bumper to bumper or horses are bucking and twisting in a nearby arena or pen.

Be sure to inform your farrier of any traumatic experiences your horse may have had that could affect his behavior during shoeing. If your horse flipped over in the crossties last week when you tried to vacuum him and has been nervous there ever since, and that is where the farrier normally works, you'd better let the farrier know.

REFLEXES

Horses are capable of quickly assuming thundering speeds from a standstill, of rising and running instantly from a lateral recumbent sleeping position and of striking or kicking in the blink of an eye. These lightning-quick reflexes have helped the horse survive for over sixty million years. The same automatic responses are what allow today's horse to perform in a vast array of spectacular events, but they also can prove to be dangerous for a farrier.

Reflexes are automatic responses to pressure on or movement of various portions of the body. The intensity of the reaction will vary depending on the horse's physical makeup (thin skin, fine haircoat, hot or cold blooded, etc.), temperament, experience, training, phys-ical restriction, degree of relaxation or tension and how forcefully and with what the pressure is applied. Each horse will react differ-ently to various levels of pressure. The reflexes of a horse that is tired, willful or resentful will be overridden. Such a horse has "tuned out" as a means of protection or defense. A nervous horse often overreacts, that is, a normal cue on the ribs to move over may cause the horse to swerve sideways 180 degrees or more. Some reflexes are interrelated or are part of a chain of reactions.

Because a horse's reflexes must be modified somewhat in order for him to be safe while he is shod, it is helpful to understand how horses learn. Behavior modifications that are based on existing instincts and reflexes cause minimal stress and result in long-lasting effects.

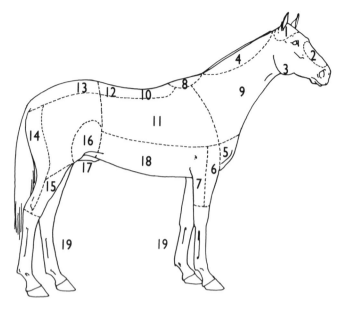

Reflex zones. From *Making Not Breaking* by Cherry Hill, Breakthrough Publishing

---

THE REACTION TO PRESSURE ON VARIOUS AREAS

1. Poll   Pressure here causes a horse to raise his head and neck and perhaps try to pull away. This reflex must be overridden.

2. Bridge of Nose   Pressure here initially causes a horse to raise his head, hollow his neck, and flip up his nose. Systematic use of a chain lead or a bosal can condition the opposite response (lower head, round neck, tuck nose).

3. Head   With no alteration in a normal neck position, an upward head extension causes forelimb flexion and hind limb extension; when the horse's head is down, hind leg flexion and foreleg extension. The parotid salivary gland is a large, long gland stretching from the base of the ear to the throat. When the head and neck posture is up and flexed, the gland is stimulated to produce saliva.

4. Crest   Touching here causes a horse to lower his neck.

5. Breast   Pressure here causes the horse to back up if the horse's head is low. If the horse's head is high, the backing reflex tends to be blocked.

6. Forelimb Extensors   Pressure on the muscles at the front of the foreleg causes the cannon and hoof to swing forward.

7. Forelimb Flexors   Pressure on the muscles at the back of the foreleg causes the knee to bend.

8. Withers   Light pressure causes the horse to lower his head, reach with his neck and nibble if he is scratched. Heavy pressure causes him to evade the pain, possibly with threatening gestures with his head and neck.

9. Neck   The neck contracts on the side where it is touched. With no alteration in normal head position, hollowing of the neck to one side induces hind leg flexion and foreleg extension on that side; a rounding of the neck results in foreleg flexion and hind leg extension on that side.

10. Back   Light pressure on the spine from the withers to the lumbosacral junction will cause the horse to hollow his back. Light pressure on one side, the left for example, will cause the spine to curve away from the pressure and move the left hind leg forward.

11. Ribs   When the horse's head is turned toward you, pressure on the ribs causes him to flex his ribs away from the pressure; his hind leg on the same side also flexes, while the opposite hind extends, causing sway or crossing.

12. Loin   Pressure causes the back to flatten or round.

13. Croup   Pressure causes the horse to tuck his tail and hindquarters and round his back.

14. Semitendinosus (Hamstrings)   Pressure causes the horse to raise his leg and/or kick backward.

15. Gaskin   Pressure causes hock flexion.

16. Flank   Pressure causes the horse to reach his hind leg forward or cow kick.

17. Sheath   Pressure may cause the horse to flex both hind legs and drop the croup.

18. Abdominals   Depending on the horse's back reaction, pressure on the abdominals can result in a contraction of the horse's belly, a rounding of the back, a lowering of the croup, an arching of the neck and perhaps a lowering and reaching forward with the neck.

19. Lower Limbs   Upward withdrawal by flexion of joints.

20. Subcutaneous Muscle   The sheet of muscle under the skin of the major mass of the body reacts to light stroking with rapid repeated twitching; firm, steady pressure causes tonic contraction.

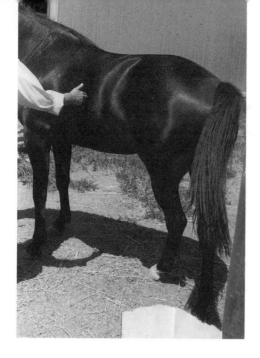

*Teach your horse to move
away from light pressure.*

In some cases, you must work with a horse's reflexes and in some instances you must completely override them. In addition to utilizing the withdrawal reflex to get a horse to pick up his foot as previously described, employ the aid of other reflexive responses. To more easily persuade an inexperienced foal to pick up his left hind foot, an assistant can activate the appropriate reflexes by turning the foal's head to the left. The left hind leg will tend to flex, thereby aiding the lifting of the left hind foot. Lifting the left fore foot can be induced by a right head turn, but this time the neck is curled slightly downward by hand pressure on the nose.

Once a horse has picked up his foot, and this is especially true with the hinds, allow the honest horse to rebalance, if necessary, or to stretch and relax before you go to work on the hoof. This only takes a few seconds and allows the horse to stand more comfortably.

When you need to reposition a horse, again use reflex principles to your advantage. For example, to move a horse's hindquarters, apply pressure to his side. He will try to move his head toward you, flex his ribs away from you and step with his hind legs away from you. Knowing this, you can set him up ahead of time in a position that makes it easier for him to do the right thing. Tip his nose toward you and then apply pressure on the ribs. (If a horse is tied in such a fashion that he can't tip his nose toward you, he will likely "lock up" and not move at all.) Horses tend to move away from light, intermittent pressure and lean into heavy steady pressure. So instead of planting a rigid fist in the horse's side, use a tapping motion with your fingers and you are likely to get better results.

Contrary to what is often seen practiced, a horse backs up naturally and more willingly from light, intermittent pressure on the points of the chest and shoulder (providing the head and neck are lowered) than by grabbing the halter and tugging on the noseband. Pressure on the bridge of the nose actually causes the untrained horse to raise his nose, hollow his back and resist backing. However, a horse can be conditioned to lower his head by applying pressure simultaneously to the poll and the nose.

The reflexes of the relaxed horse are not on edge. Therefore, he may be a bit slower to respond to your cues but also less likely to resist or explode. If you intend to work on one hoof for an extended period of time, work on level ground and make sure that the horse's other three legs are in a balanced configuration. Older horses may be stiff, especially in the hind joints, and may be more comfortable and cooperative if you hold their legs lower than usual.

Be aware of accidental cues or conflicting signals you may be giving a horse as you work around his legs. Is your hair or your hat tickling his abdominals or his ribs, setting off reflex contractions? Are you inadvertently applying pressure on the coronary band as you bring the foot forward to mimic the farrier's position when he uses a hoof stand? Is your horse covered with reflex-triggering flies? Be sure to use fly repellent when necessary and train your horse to stand still for spraying well before your farrier's visit.

As you teach your horse to stand still for longer periods of time, keep a specific goal in mind: for example, standing still on two hind legs and one front leg for two minutes. Remember to

- Pick the best foundation behavior to build on. If a foal stands quietly alongside the wall of the box stall with its dam nearby, begin here. Don't mix weaning, the first tying lesson and trimming into one exciting catastrophe!
- Reward all attempts the horse makes to achieve the behavior you want. At the beginning, require the foal to hold up the leg for fifteen seconds at a time. Let the leg down only when the foal is standing quietly and not struggling. Give a scratch on the withers as added show of approval.
- Don't go too fast toward the goal. Be realistic about how long a young or an unconditioned horse should be required to stand. If the horse is honestly tired or uncomfortable, give him a break. Don't risk losing the rapport you are developing with a young horse by asking him to stand an inordinate amount of time.
- Don't get stuck in one particular stage. If your goal is for your farrier to be able to drive and wring six nails and set the clinches before putting the foot down, don't expect him to break this pro-

cess up into two or more segments for more than one or two shoe-ings or the horse may expect this permanently (and you might be searching for another farrier).

One of the most dangerous times in shoeing a horse is when the farrier has just finished driving a nail, but has yet to wring off the tip. At that point, the unpredictable behavior of some horses may result in them suddenly jerking their foot away from the farrier, possibly causing injury to the shoer or the horse from the protruding nail tip. It is imperative that all horses have manners and respect for the shoeing process.

If you have an older horse that missed "the basics," take him to a well-respected professional trainer who specializes in ground manners. Most horses that have had proper handling as young horses take their first shoeing "in stride" and actually appear to enjoy their time with the farrier.

Foal Hoof Management

Raising a foal so that he has the best chance of exhibiting optimum athletic performance as an adult requires careful attention. Your foal's hoof management program should be a combined effort between you, your farrier and your veterinarian (Chapter 16). Trimming should be designed in light of your foal's present configuration as well as his anticipated adult conformation.

Unless you are very experienced in raising foals and know your foal is normal, you should arrange for a veterinary examination the day after birth. This will allow your veterinarian to evaluate the foal's limbs and determine whether any deviations are normal or whether they will require close observation or treatment. Most angular deformities greater than 15 degrees require immediate veterinary treatment; however, the majority of foals do not fall into this category.

A foal is born with soft feathers of horn on the bottom of its hooves. These wear off by the end of a normal first day. The texture of the baby (neonate) hoof is cornified, yet soft and waxy. It remains somewhat that way the first week but gradually hardens to more durable hoof horn. The last bit of neonate hoof will have grown down to ground level by about six months of age.

A regular program of farrier care should begin when the foal is about one month old. Rasping, if even necessary, should be very minimal. Radical rasping or trimming usually does more harm than good with the very young foal. Closure of the growth plates (physeal closure) has an important bearing on the timing of corrective treatments.

Many foals born with crooked limbs straighten without any formal treatment, and those that don't can often be corrected with care

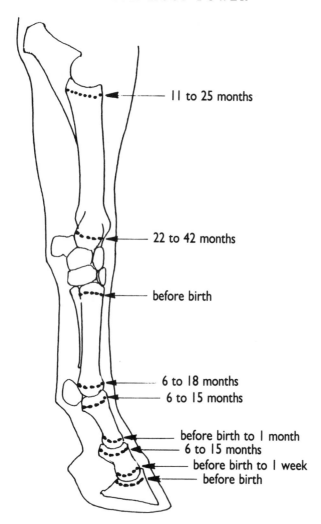

Growth plate closures

from a competent veterinarian and farrier and by proper management. For example, many foals are born knock-kneed (carpus valgus), that is, they stand with their knees closer together than their hooves.

Because most newborn foals' chests are very narrow, the front limbs are very close together at the chest. The foal, in its attempt to stabilize itself when standing and grazing, widens its base of support by increasing the distance between its hooves, which allows the lower limb to rotate outward. This causes the limbs to bend inward at the knees, bringing the knees even closer together.

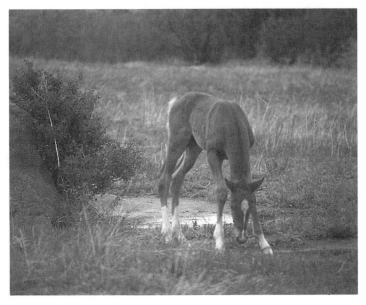

The suckling foal in a normal grazing stance

INCORRECT, "CORRECTIVE" TRIMMING

If the hooves of a knock-kneed, toed-out foal are aggressively altered by rasping, it may be possible to make the limbs appear "ideal," but in reality they are probably headed for a lifetime of problems. Some outdated corrective trimming principles are dangerous for foals. One procedure used to correct a toed-out individual was to rotate the toe of the hoof capsule forward by lowering the outside hoof wall to make it shorter than the inside wall. In addition, a half shoe would be applied to the inside wall to further rotate the hoof to point forward. This had the effect of moving the limb underneath the horse's body and shifting more of the weight to the outside of the limb.

It has been observed that lowering the outside wall of toed-out foals before three months of age can result in a permanently bowed-out fetlock. This interrupts the natural development process and places abnormal stresses on portions of the growth plate. As the limbs compensate and remodel in response to the uneven weight imposed on them, they form a sloped growth plate rather than a desirable horizontal configuration.

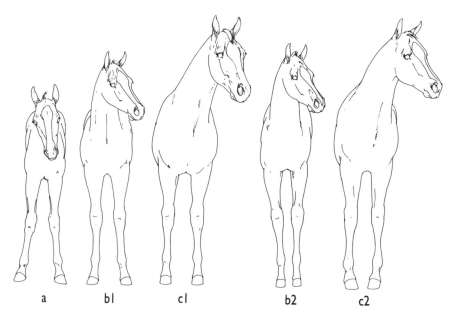

a   b1   c1   b2   c2

Correct and incorrect foal trimming
a. Suckling foal
b1. Weanling allowed to toe-out normally (correct)
b2. Weanling trimmed to stand straight (incorrect)
c1. This is b1 as a yearling, now straight (correct)
c2. This is b2 as a yearling, now toed-in (incorrect)

Impatience to "correct" a normally knock-kneed, fetlock-rotated-out foal by lowering the outside wall can also result in sheared heels. Such a problem usually doesn't occur if the hoof is kept in ML balance and the foal's own development is allowed to correct the knock-kneed condition. Therefore, it is generally recommended to *not* lower the outside wall on knock-kneed, fetlock-rotated-out foals under three months of age. Because a knock-kneed foal tends to break over to the inside of the hoof center, squaring the toe will encourage a more central breakover and help maintain ML balance.

KNEE AND CHEST CONFORMATION

Depending on chest conformation, a foal will usually be somewhat knock-kneed until six to eight months of age. The tighter (more narrow) the chest, the more the face of the knee will naturally (and

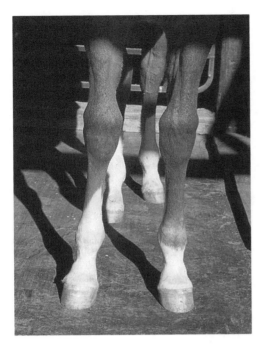

The same foal at four months

should be allowed to) rotate around. The fetlocks also face outward somewhat to allow horizontal formation and maintenance of the growth plates. Incorrect "corrective" trimming to force the fetlock and hoof to face forward often results in a sheared fetlock that no longer hinges perpendicular to the limb. When this happens, as the foal matures it often will attain a toed-in stance.

At eight to ten months of age, the normal widening of the foal's chest tends to move the front limbs away from the body, allowing the knees and fetlocks to straighten and rotate inward so they are more directly under the body mass in a straight column. With foals that have been improperly altered, the limbs rotate inward as the chest widens, until the lower limbs and hooves start pointing toward each other. Knock-kneed foals that have the genetics for heavy bodies and wide chests especially should not be trimmed early or aggressively for their knock-kneed, toed-out condition, or by the time their chests widen they may become bowlegged.

The foal that has mild to moderate knock-knees, if kept level and balanced through his growing months, will stand relatively straight as a yearling because his legs rotate inward with age and weight gain.

The foal whose limb from the elbow down is rotated outward is not so lucky. Very little can be done to change this conformational defect. If such a foal is kept level and balanced and if the foal develops

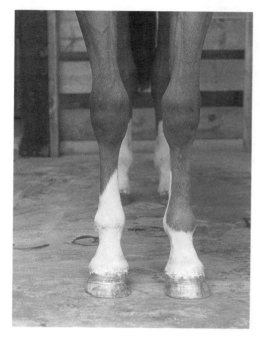

The same horse at ten months

a sufficient chest, he may become an acceptable athlete, although he may tend to interfere and have an odd walk the rest of his life. If this foal is mistakenly treated for bowed-in fetlocks and his foot is made to face forward when he is young, then he *will* have a problem as an adult, a toed-in foot with a rotated-out limb.

REGULAR FARRIER CARE

Besides assessing the static balance of your foal's hooves in relation to his limbs, your farrier will evaluate the foal's hoof-wear patterns. In most cases, rasping required to balance a hoof is done conservatively and with close monitoring of the natural wear. By squaring the toe, a hoof can be encouraged to break over at the center. By checking for evenness and symmetry, the farrier can evaluate the natural tendency of the fetlock, pastern and hoof to align with the cannon. With the foal's front limb flexed at the knee, the farrier lets the dorsal surface of the cannon rest in the palm of his hand. The fetlock and hoof are allowed to fall into their normal axis at rest. The farrier can then evaluate the heels for evenness, the relationship of the hoof to the limb and the symmetry of the frog in relation to the hoof.

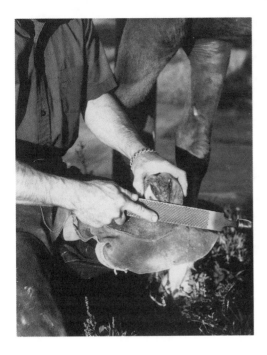

Lightly rasping the foal's hoof

BONE DEVELOPMENT PROBLEMS

A number of factors predispose the growing horse to alterations in bone development. Rapid growth, trauma to the growth plates or cartilage, genetic predisposition and nutritional imbalances or a combination of two or more of these factors may increase the incidence or severity of the problem.

The major nutritional imbalances that appear to be related to developmental disorders of the muscles and skeleton in the growing horse are a deficiency or excess of energy, protein, calcium, phosphorus, zinc, and vitamins D and A, and a deficiency of copper and possibly manganese. The principal effect of these imbalances is an interference with bone formation that can result in malformations, including angular limb deformities and acquired flexion deformities.

Rapid growth appears to be the primary factor, and it is prompted by a horse's genetic predisposition, high-energy intake and feeding for maximum growth after a period of stunting. Not providing adequate amounts of properly formulated creep feed to a suckling and then providing an excess of feed following weaning can result in a growth spurt that leads to flexure problems.

Greater trauma occurs to the growth plates of a foal of excess body weight. The excess weight is concentrated on growth plates and joint cartilage surfaces that are proportionally small, and alterations in bone formations can result. Horses with short, upright pasterns and those breeds that are faster growing, larger and finer-boned are affected more frequently.

Nutritional imbalances may lead to problems. Excess dietary energy from the intake of large amounts of grain results in rapid growth, which triggers alterations in bone formation that can cause poor bone quality. To prevent this problem, a good rule of thumb is to feed a *maximum* of 1 pound of concentrate per day for each month of age up to a maximum of 8 to 9 pounds daily. Often much less than this is appropriate, depending on hay fed and type of pasture available. (Confer with your veterinarian and refer to the Recommended Reading list in the Appendix.)

Inadequate quantity or quality of protein in the ration interferes with proper bone growth and development and can decrease the growth rate. Feeding excess protein, however, does not increase the growth rate above that achieved when requirements are just met. And increasing protein without adequate minerals such as calcium and phosphorus to support the faster growth rate can lead to bone development problems. The recommended protein content of the ration should be met and not exceeded by more than 2%. In the total ration, the dry matter protein percentage that is recommended is 18% for nursing foals, 16% for weanlings, 13% for yearlings, and 10% for 2-year-olds. It may be necessary to utilize a supplement to ensure the growing horse is receiving essential amino acids (see Resource Guide in the Appendix).

The growing horse must have adequate amounts of available (capable of being absorbed) calcium and phosphorus. The phosphorus present in grains, wheat bran and other concentrates is less available to the horse than the phosphorus in roughages and minerals. Excess phosphorus can decrease calcium absorption. Excess calcium can decrease absorption of trace minerals.

Providing that the *amount* of calcium and phosphorus are adequate, the *ratio* of Ca:P in the ration of the growing horse can range from 0.8:1 to 3:1 and in the mature horse from 0.8:1 to 8:1 without problems. If the amount of either calcium or phosphorus is inadequate or the ratio is outside these limits, alterations in bone formation may occur.

The most common feeding practices that are responsible for nutritional imbalances in the growing horse are feeding too much grain, feeding alfalfa hay without adding phosphorus to the ration, or feeding a grain mix that is inadequate in calcium, phosphorus and protein when grass hay is fed (Chapter 14).

To treat problems resulting from alterations in bone formation, alfalfa and grain are removed from the diet and as much good-quality grass hay as the horse will eat is provided. The lower energy and protein content slows the growth rate and allows recovery to occur. However, grass hay is usually deficient in both calcium and phosphorus, so 4 ounces of 12:12 Ca:P mineral mix must be fed daily. It can be mixed with a minimal amount of grain containing molasses to keep the mineral from settling out.

Although exercise is often detrimental for cases of acute angular deformities, it is usually beneficial for treatment of flexion deformities. The normally developing horse should be allowed free-choice exercise (Chapter 14).

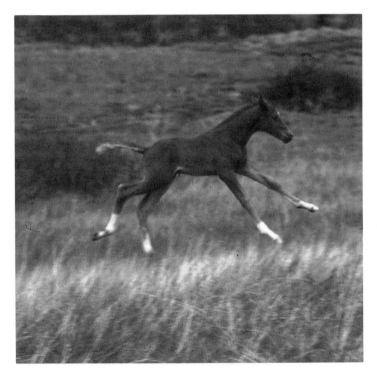

The suckling foal enjoying free exercise

Horsekeeping

Proper horse management encompasses design and maintenance of facilities, sanitation, exercise, nutrition and routine care. These subjects are covered in their entirety in other books (see Recommended Reading in the Appendix), so here we will focus on those points that directly affect hoof quality and health.

If you follow good management practices, your horse will have a better chance of living a healthy, safe and comfortable life; he will be more able to give you an optimum performance, and you both will enjoy his longer active life.

FACILITIES

Your horse's living quarters, whether stall, pasture or paddock, should have well-drained footing.

The Barn Site

The site for your barn should be properly prepared so that the soil and other materials beneath the floor percolate well. Ideally, the finished level of the barn site should be 8 to 12 inches above ground level. If the existing soil is well drained, the site can be prepared by the addition of 6 inches of crushed rock covered by soil. Pure clay (a traditional favorite) does not percolate well. Soil blends or synthetic materials (depending on locale) might work as well or better than clay for site preparation.

A site with poorly-drained soils requires excavation to between 3 and 10 feet. Several feet of large rock should be laid at the base of the excavation. Crushed rock of decreasing sizes should follow in layers, leaving about 1 foot for the site's topsoil. A mixture of clay, sand or other materials (such as road base or some small gravels) usually works well.

Stall Flooring

The stall flooring is the layer added on top of the prepared site. Factors to consider when choosing flooring include initial cost, longevity, maintenance, cushion, drainage, odor retention, ease of cleaning and sanitizing, and traction. Be sure to consider the type of bedding you plan to use, as some flooring/bedding conditions are undesirable.

For box stalls, the tamped clay floor has been a traditional favorite because it provides cushion and good traction, and is warm and quiet. Tamped clay does not drain well, so clay stalls must be sloped to allow drainage. In addition, urine pools can create large potholes, requiring the clay floor to be leveled routinely and overhauled annually.

Mixtures of clay and sand or clay and crushed rock are usually readily available and will have improved drainage over pure clay while retaining most of the desirable features of the clay floor. Road base is often such a mixture—a blend of crushed limestone and clay. But while a road-base blend may result in better sanitation, it tends to be unstable under a horse's movement. As a consequence, it can become mixed in with the bedding, be ingested with the feed, and be a pawing horse's delight. Having an extra stall in your barn and rotating horses so one stall can rest at all times will minimize floor maintenance.

Concrete makes a permanent, low-maintenance floor that is fairly easy to sanitize, but it requires very deep bedding because it can be hard, cold and abrasive. A barefoot pawing horse can severely damage his hooves on a concrete floor. Concrete floors must be designed with a drain or a slope and should have a textured surface to ensure good traction.

Asphalt (blacktop) is a relatively permanent material that has some give, is nonslip and is not as cold as concrete. It too is abrasive, requires deep bedding and initially is one of the most costly choices.

"Rubber" stall mats are usually a combination of rubber, clay, nylon, and rayon. They act as an intermediary between the soil and the bedding. They have superior cushioning, which makes them comfortable. Mats can be easily sanitized, make stall cleaning easy, decrease dust so horses stay cleaner and decrease the amount of bedding required up to 50 percent. They also prevent a pawing horse from digging holes in the stall. Stall mats are expensive at the outset, and if they are not properly texturized, they can be slippery.

Interlocking plastic stall grids are designed to be installed with sand or road base. The large holes and spaces in the grids are filled with sand, providing a tough floor with good drainage. If properly installed, such a floor is impervious to a pawing horse.

Wood, an old-time favorite for tie stalls, is really not appropriate for box stalls. Although it is warmer than concrete and fairly durable if treated wood is used, it can be slippery, difficult to sanitize and deodorize and noisy under a nervous horse.

Bedding

Bedding should be easy to handle, absorbent and comfortable. The bedding with the highest water-absorbing capacity, however, is not necessarily best. An extremely absorbent bedding sops up too much urine, and if the bedding is not changed frequently, the horse's hooves will be subjected to constant wetness. On the other hand, a bedding with very little absorbency lets too much moisture pass through to the flooring and can result in pooling. The ideal bedding in most cases has a moderate absorbency and is free from dust, mold and injurious substances.

Hardwood products are generally undesirable for bedding because of their poor absorbency and in some cases, such as with black walnut, their toxicity. Horses merely coming in contact with such shavings have experienced founder and death. Wheat straw, because of its high glaze, does not become as slimy and sloppy as oat straw when wet and is less palatable to horses than oat straw, so it may be safer to use with the horse that overeats. Barley straw should be avoided because of the sharp, barbed awns that can become lodged in a horse's gums. Straw of any kind is very slippery on wood floors. All beddings, even peat moss, have the potential to be dusty. Dusty bedding material should be avoided to prevent respiratory problems in the horse.

Farrier Work Area

An important part of your facilities is an all-weather, level, well-lighted work area for your farrier. Specific recommendations are given in Chapter 16.

SANITATION

Sanitation practices are essential for your horse's hoof health. Sanitation involves proper management of manure, flies and moisture. A 1,000-pound horse produces approximately 50 pounds of manure per day and from 6 to 10 gallons of urine, which when soaked up by bedding, can constitute another 50 pounds.

Urine breaks down into products that contain ammonia, which produces a pungent vapor that is injurious to the eyes and lungs. The combination of dung and urine is a perfect medium for the proliferation of bacteria, which can begin destructive processes on hoof horn. When certain fecal bacteria ferment, their secretions can dissolve the intertubular "hoof cement." Moist manure softens, loosens and encourages the breakdown of hoof horn cells.

Wherever there is manure, there are parasite larvae and flies. Proper management of manure the best way to break the parasite life cycle and control the fly population. Manure should be collected daily and hauled away, spread immediately on a pasture or arena, or stored for later distribution. Some refuse collection services accept manure.

Hydrated lime is used to "sweeten" stall floors and pens, as it lowers the acidity of the urine in the stall. It also causes the dirt particles to clump, which allows air to more easily get at and penetrate the wet soil, thereby drying it.

MOISTURE CONTROL

By now you know that making a horse stand in mud is often the very worst thing you could do. And that hoof dressing should not be indiscriminately slathered on your horse's hooves to "moisturize" them. Since the modern riding horse evolved on semiarid plains, the healthy hoof is designed to be dry and hard. Your role as manager of your horse in confinement is to provide an environment that allows the hoof to be dry, hard and healthy.

If your horse is getting adequate exercise and the footing of his stall, pen or pasture is well drained, the moisture balance between the inner and outer layers of his hooves probably remains at a relatively constant, healthy level. If your horse stands inactive for long periods of time, sufficient moisture may not be delivered via the blood to the hoof, and his hoof walls may tend to contract. But if his hooves are too soft from mud, frequent baths or excessive hoof dressing, they contain too much moisture, and the hoof spreads and the layers separate.

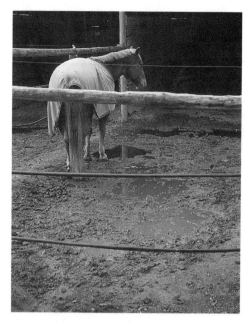

Mud can be devastating to hooves.

The effects of repeated wet/dry conditions can be devastating to hooves. Hoof conditions worsen during hot, humid weather, especially when horses are turned out at night in dew-laden pastures and then are either left out where the sun will dry the hooves or are put in a stall where the bedding dries the hooves. Horses who receive daily baths or rinses or those that repeatedly walk through mud and then stand in the sun experience a similar decay in hoof quality. In both cases, the hoof is going through a stressful moisture expansion/contraction that is damaging to the hoof structures.

If you want a "first hand" example of this drying-out process, poke your fingernails into some fresh mud and then let the mud dry. Your nails and cuticles may begin to split and crack after just one episode.

In the process of drying out, the hoof develops cracks, and the cracks are packed with mud so they continue getting larger and spreading. In addition, the cellular cement that holds the hoof horn together breaks down. The result is a frayed pulpy mass of fibrous tubules. Drying mud and water also leach out essential nutrients and oils that are responsible for maintaining hoof flexibility.

Follow these guidelines to maintain your horse's hooves at an optimum, constant moisture level:

- Keep stalls dry.
- Provide turnout areas that are not muddy.
- Minimize bathing.

- Minimize wet-dry episodes such as hosing legs and then putting the horse in a stall with dry sawdust bedding.
- Closely monitor the moisture balance in hooves that must wear full pads for an extended period of time.
- Use hoof dressing discriminately.
- Use a hoof sealer when appropriate, such as during the wet seasons, if the horse must be bathed frequently, if the hooves show signs of surface cracks or if your farrier has rasped the wall of the hoof to shape it during trimming.

The hoof has two natural protective coverings, the periople and the stratum tectorium, which retard moisture movement from either direction—from the outside environment into the hoof or from the inner layer of the hoof to the outside. When the thin layer of stratum tectorium is rasped away, application of a sealer is recommended.

Because a healthy, strong hoof is naturally dry and hard, many farriers recommend not applying grease or oil that softens the hoof. About the only time hoof dressing is warranted is when the bulbs of the heels have become so dry that they are beginning to crack. In order to restore their pliability, rub a product containing animal fat (such as lanolin or fish oil) into the heels daily until the desired result has been achieved. It is thought that petroleum-based products may emulsify the hoof's natural oils and actually remove moisture.

EXERCISE

Exercise is essential for maintaining overall health and for the proper development of bones and dense, tough hooves. All horses of all ages need exercise every day, either a ride or a minimum turnout of two hours in a large pen or pasture.

Exercise's many benefits include assistance in the development and repair of tissue. It can improve the quality and strength of bones, tendons, ligaments and hooves. Regular, moderate stress creates dense, stress-resistant bone and hooves. Exercise also conditions and stretches muscles and tendons, resulting in less chance of injury and lameness.

It is important that any exercise area is safely fenced and free from hazardous objects. Footing should not be excessively deep. Hyperextension of the fetlock in deep sand can do permanent damage to tendons. Rocky footing can encourage the development of dense, tough hooves but can also cause hoof damage, especially if the horse's hooves are weak and vulnerable when he is first turned out in a rocky pasture.

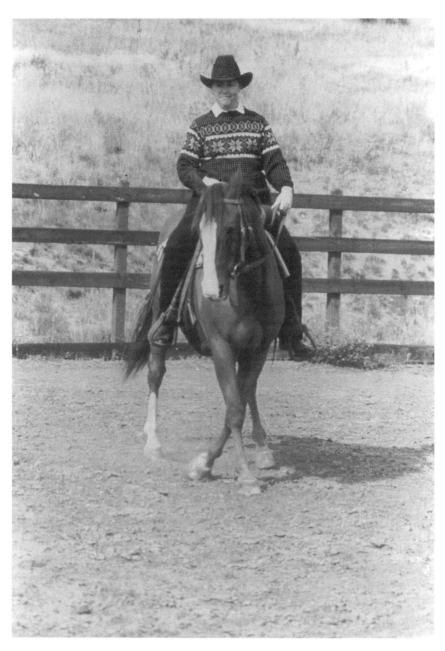

Riding can provide enjoyable, varied exercise. Cherry Hill on Zinger

Riding is an ideal way to provide daily exercise for a horse (and rider!), as it can be controlled yet varied. Free exercise is the least labor intensive and most natural way of providing exercise. However, many horses turned out do not self-exercise and will probably spend most of their time eating if the turnout area is a pasture.

Ponying is a good choice in an arena or in open spaces on varied terrain. Ponying a young horse on the surface that he will be worked on when he is an adult provides an opportunity for specialized adaptation of tissues.

Longeing is an option best suited to horses over two years of age. Because of repeated, uneven loading of the limbs associated with circle work, younger horses may suffer strain from excessive longeing. For any age horse, it is ideal if the longe circle is at least 20 meters, or 66 feet in diameter.

Electric horse walkers are useful for warm-ups and occasional exercise sessions but should not be viewed as the mainstay of a horse's exercise program. Thirty minutes of walking once or twice a week is a good alternative if on those days the horse would otherwise have to stand in a stall. Depending entirely on a walker for exercise, however, can encourage undesirable habits such as a stiff carriage, resistance, laziness and boredom.

A treadmill can be used for an occasional workout, providing the horse is gradually conditioned to the work and carefully monitored for signs of stress. A continuous climb at the 5- to 7-degree slope characteristic of most treadmills is extremely fatiguing. A workout using a treadmill is accomplished in about half the time required for most other forms of exercise. Treadmills are used successfully for muscle development, particularly in the forearm, chest, stifle and gaskin areas. However, a treadmill workout could be devastating to the tendons of a horse with long toes (Chapter 5 and 11).

NUTRITION

Feeding horses is a complex topic (see Recommended Reading in the Appendix). The following nutrition guidelines relate specifically to the health of the horse's hooves.

- Know each horse's feed requirements. Don't assume that commercial feeds or hays provide all that a horse needs. Several important nutrients that are necessary for high-quality hooves are frequently deficient in horses' rations (see Resource Guide in the Appendix).

- Know exactly what you are feeding. Read and understand the feed tags of commercially prepared feed. If you buy large batches of hay consistent in type and quality, ask your county extension agent how to have your hay tested for its nutrient content. Otherwise, use hay composition guidelines listed in the Appendix.
- Monitor your horse's weight routinely to determine the amount of feed required, to prevent obesity and to minimize the chance of laminitis. Use a weight tape, scale or the accompanying chart to determine your horse's approximate weight. One hundred extra

Heart Girth in Inches	Weight in Pounds
54	492
56	531
58	596
60	664
62	722
64	785
66	852
68	902
70	985
72	1065
74	1220
76	1265

pounds of body weight plus 200 pounds of tack and rider can be very harmful to your horse's feet and limbs.
- Know exactly how much you are feeding. Weigh hay at each feeding. Flakes (also called fleks, leaves, slabs, or slices) can vary from 2 to 7 pounds, depending on the type of hay, moisture content, how tightly the hay was baled and the adjustment on the baler for flake thickness. Feed hay at an approximate rate of 1½ to 1¾ pounds per 100 pounds of body weight. A 1,000-pound horse will require about 15 to 17½ pounds of hay per day.
- Feed grain to young, growing horses, horses in hard work and lactating broodmares. Grain should be fed by weight, not volume. Feed by the pound, not by the scoop or by the quart. Oats are much lighter than corn, so a quart of oats will weigh far less than a quart of corn. The weight of a quart of some of the grains commonly fed

to horses is as follows: bran, ½ pound; oats, 1 pound; barley, 1½ pounds; corn 1¾ pounds.

- It should be determined how much additional energy a horse requires beyond the energy provided by the hay he receives. Energy is expressed as Total Digestible Nutrients (TDN) or Digestible Energy (DE). The energy values of grains vary greatly. The TDN in oats is approximately 65%; barley is 72%; and corn is 85%. This means that a pound of corn contains nearly a third more energy than a pound of oats.

- Make changes in feed gradually over a period of a week or so. When increasing or decreasing grain, makes the changes in ½-pound increments. Feed the new amount for several days before making the next adjustment.

- When turning a horse out to pasture for the first time, be sure the horse has had a full feed of hay. Limit grazing to one-half hour for the first two days. Then one-half hour twice a day for two days, then one hour twice a day and so on. Keep a close watch on horses that are on pasture, as they can quickly become overweight or suffer laminitis (Chapter 11), a debilitating, life-threatening condition often caused from too much rich or green feed.

- Be sure it is impossible for a horse to get into the feed room. Horses do not know when to stop eating and can literally "eat themselves to death." An excess amount of grain can cause colic or laminitis.

- Do not feed a horse immediately after hard work and do not work a horse until at least one hour after a full feeding. The horse's digestive system is sensitive and must be considered when planning work requirements before and after meals.

- Feed the highest-quality hay you can find. Learn what makes good-quality hay (see Recommended Reading in the Appendix) and take the time to shop around before buying.

- Balance your horses' rations by providing free-choice trace mineralized salt. Trace mineralized salt contains sodium, chloride and usually iodine, zinc, iron, manganese, copper and cobalt.

- Depending on the horse's age and type of feed, determine if calcium and phosphorus need to be supplemented and in what ratio. If calcium is deficient, limestone can be added to the grain. If phosphorus is low, monosodium phosphate can be used as a source. If both calcium and phosphorus are low, di-calcium phosphate can be used. Blocks are available that provide trace mineralized salt plus calcium and phosphorus in various ratios. Beware of feeding excess phosphorus (in the form of bran or a supplement), as it can have a negative effect on the Ca:P ration and result in abnormal hoof horn structure.

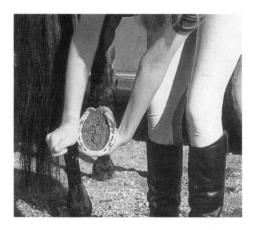

Pick out the hooves before riding.

- After formulating the hay and grain portion of your horse's ration, choose a hoof supplement that provides any missing nutrients. Frequently hooves (and haircoat) benefit from the addition of DL-methionine, lysine, calcium, biotin and other substances to the ration (see Resource Guide in the Appendix).

DAILY INSPECTION ROUTINE

Horses are creatures of habit and respond well to good management practices that follow a regular pattern. Establishing daily, weekly, monthly and yearly routines will increase your horse's well-being and minimize your veterinary bills.

You should develop a habit of looking at your horses so that in a couple of moments you can determine their overall health. First you must have a good sense of what is normal for horses in general and for each of your own horses. Like humans, horses can exhibit a wide range of characteristics, and each horse will have his own set of norms.

Your routine examination (which can occur at each feeding) should include noting your horse's overall stance and attitude, the condition of his legs, how he moves and clues in his living area. If you notice a difference in his legs or hooves, halter your horse and bring him to an area where you can give him a thorough visual check and palpation. So that you have a baseline for comparison in relation to texture, temperature, and sensitivity of your horse's legs and hooves, be sure to carry out a preliminary examination when everything appears normal (see Recommended Reading in the Appendix).

Suggested Hoof Examination Routine

- Notice which leg he is resting.
- Notice if his front legs are both ahead of or behind their normal (vertical) configuration.
- Notice if his hind legs are ahead of or behind their normal configuration.
- Notice if he is reluctant to walk to the examination area.
- Wipe any mud or manure off the hoof wall and coronet.
- Pick out all of his hooves.
- Note any sensitivity in the clefts of frog (including the central cleft) when using a hoof pick to clean them.
- Look for imbedded rocks, splinters, nails, etc., in any part of the hoof, including the coronet.
- Test each branch of the shoe to see if it is loose.
- Sight down the bottom surface of the shoe to see if it is still flat. Sometimes the heel of a shoe will be stepped on and bent down and go unnoticed because it is still tight.
- Note if the shoe has slipped or twisted off to one side.
- Note if the shoe has slipped backward. (Be careful not to confuse this with a shoe that has purposely been set back by your farrier.)
- Check the clinches to see if they are tight or if they have opened up and started to pull through the hoof.
- Look for signs of injury on the coronary band, bulbs or lower leg.

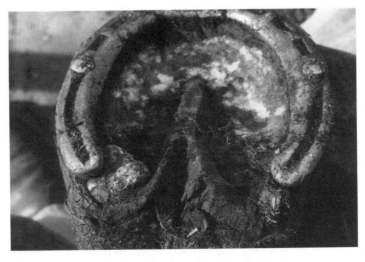

Rock wedged under shoe heel

The Lost Shoe Dilemma

Lost shoes are an inconvenience for both the rider and the farrier and can cause hoof wall damage. Damage can occur traumatically when the shoe is first lost or later as the unprotected hoof wears and breaks. It doesn't take long for the DP and ML balance of a shoeless hoof to be affected.

If a horse loses a shoe soon after he is shod, it is likely due to him stepping on the shoe or getting it caught on something. If a horse loses a shoe later in the shoeing period, it may be due to worn nail heads or loosening clinches. Most lost shoes are front shoes.

Not all horses lose shoes. In a study that spanned a three-year period, one farrier documented that 80 percent of all lost shoes were attributed to 20 percent of the horses. And certain horses in that 20-percent group lost most of the shoes. One client's gelding lost more shoes in one year than another client's four horses lost together in over ten years! The average shoe loss in this study was 1.33 shoes per horse per year. Lost shoes can be caused by a variety of hoof-related factors, including a horse's conformation, way of going, poor riding, deep or wet footing and poor management (Chapters 8 and 9).

MAJOR FACTORS

Wet Environment

Excessive moisture is a principal cause of lost shoes; soft hooves simply do not hold nails securely. Farriers cringe when a wet spell descends, for they know the phone will be alive with clients distraught over lost shoes. Besides disrupting the moisture balance of the hoof, mud is accused of mechanically removing shoes. Although it is unlikely that mud can actually suck a shoe off, deep mud *can* interfere with a horse's timing and balance. The mud slows down one leg, another one comes unstuck suddenly and lands haphazardly and plucks off a shoe. (Note: Other heavy or deep footing, such as sand, snow or even long grass, can also alter limb movement and result in lost shoes.)

Hoof and Limb Conformation

A horse with very sloping front pasterns, and especially with limbs set ahead of his body and underrun heels, will require front shoes placed so far back on his hoof (for flexor tendon support) that the shoe could easily be stepped on. Treatment for underrun heels include using a shoe with a very generous base of support at the heels, which can easily be stepped on (Chapters 5 and 11). In an attempt to minimize repeated lost shoes, the heel support may be compromised but then the underrun heel condition has a diminished chance of correction. Many farriers recommend that a horse with extended heels or egg bar shoes on the fronts receive only controlled exercise (riding, longeing, driving), since free exercise often results in these shoes being lost.

The base-narrow, toed-out horse may step off a front shoe with the other front foot. The downhill horse (withers lower than hips) and the short-backed, long-legged horse are both "set up" to overreach. Horses with poor-quality hooves, thin hoof walls, and shelly horn often lose shoes simply because their hoof is too weak to hold the clinches.

Overdue Shoeing

Leaving shoes on too long is a common cause of lost shoes. When a shoe is not reset in a timely manner, the hoof will overgrow the shoe at the heels and quarters. The small edge of hoof wall that is left to support the horse's weight collapses and the shoe is forced up into the hoof, frequently becoming imbedded in the sole. This crushing of the hoof wall is a cause of underrun heels, and the pressure on the sole is a cause of corns and abscesses. Once the hoof collapses over the shoe, the nails are then too long and the loose clinches work on the nail

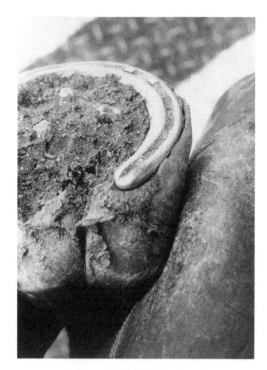

Shoe imbedded in hoof

holes, making them larger. The loose nails then get sheared off or the shoe rotates on the hoof and gets stepped off.

When a shoe is left on too long, even if it remains tightly attached, the hoof grows out of balance (LT-LH), which can result in a delayed breakover and lost shoes because of overreaching.

Good Shoeing

It is ironical that the better a horse is shod, the greater the chances are of his losing a shoe. A farrier's number one priority can either be to keep a shoe on at all costs or to shoe the horse for balance, support and long-term soundness. These two goals never coincide; it is one or the other. A good shoeing job does not consist of a close fit around the entire edge of the hoof with very little shoe visible and eight heavy nails with long clinches holding the shoe on very securely. A shoe that is fit full with proper support will have more steel exposed at the quarters and heels, which may make it more likely to be stepped on.

Shoes with eight nails and long clinches resist the forces of a horse that has snagged a shoe. The long clinches do not open up easily and can pull large hunks of hoof wall away with them when the horse finally does wrench the shoe off. Now the horse may have two problems: a sprained joint and extensive hoof damage.

If a horse steps on his shoe or gets it caught in wire, it is better for the shoe to come off cleanly than for the horse to damage his hoof or limb because the shoe was on too securely. Therefore, the nails used should be high-quality slim nails with thin shanks. The clinches should be relatively small, about ⅛ inch square, and very smooth, so when a shoe does get caught, the clinches open up easily and slide cleanly through the nail holes in the hoof wall.

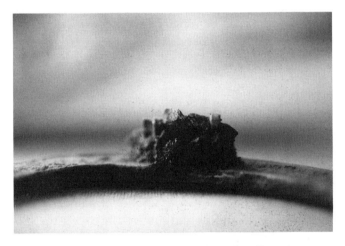

The shoe may take a chunk of hoof wall with it.

Miscellaneous

Other reasons why shoes are lost include alteration in stride because of traction devices and unusual one-time circumstances: the horse paws a wire fence, takes a misstep in his pen or stall, steps on himself while backing out of a trailer, or gets stepped on by another horse's shoe, for example, during a polo match. In certain circumstances, such as with long-distance horses, new shoes and nails wear out and come off before the hoof is ready to be trimmed. Infrequent exercise and turnout in a very small area also result in lost shoes.

FIRST AID FOR A LOST SHOE

Even if a hoof has not been damaged by the act of losing a shoe, the hoof can quickly be chipped or bruised if not protected. A hoof that is trimmed to go barefoot has rounded edges that resist breaking and chipping, but the shod hoof has relatively sharp edges. Without the protection of a shoe, it will be very prone to damage. (This is why it is not a good idea to pull the shoes and turn the horse out before he gets a good "barefoot trim.")

When a horse has lost a shoe, the hoof should be cleaned thoroughly and either a protective boot or tape should be applied (Chapter 5). The horse should be kept in a clean, dry stall until the shoe is replaced. It is a good idea for trail riders to carry a rubber boot on rides. If a large portion of hoof is missing from the quarters where the nails were clinched, it can be repaired with prosthetic materials and shod normally, or glue-on-shoes can be applied until new hoof grows down.

PREVENTING LOST SHOES

The best way to prevent lost shoes is to have your horse regularly shod, keep his feet dry and ride him in a balanced fashion. Perhaps the simplest and most effective shoeing solution to chronic lost shoes (considering that the hooves are already balanced) is to apply squared-toe shoes on the hinds and squared or rocker toe shoes on the fronts (see figure on page 71).

Spooned-heel shoes on the front hooves can be helpful for pawing horses and chronic overreachers. From ¾ to 1 inch of the extended heels of the front shoe are bent upward until they are parallel with the heel buttresses. There must be a space of ⅛ to ¼ inch between the spooned heels and the hoof buttresses to prevent contact with the heel bulbs and/or buttresses. Heel shields (cliplike extensions welded around the edge of the shoe heels) prevent the hind shoe from grabbing the edge of the front shoe heel and pulling it off. Care must also be taken in fitting these shoes that the normal migration of the shoe forward and the dropping of the bulbs during weight bearing do not cause the heel shields to contact the heel bulbs.

Horse owners should employ a daily inspection, which includes picking out a horse's feet (Chapter 14). It is important to recognize normal hoof smell, texture and sensitivity so abnormalities can be detected. An owner should be capable of recognizing a bent shoe, a loose clinch, an overgrown hoof wall.

An occasional lost shoe is a fact of life for a shod horse. In the majority of cases, a lost shoe is not the farrier's fault, so there is no reason to directly or indirectly blame the farrier. Shoes do not just "fall" off, nor does a horse "throw" a shoe. Usually a shoe comes off because the horse steps on it or catches it on something or because the horse's hooves are too wet or overdue for shoeing.

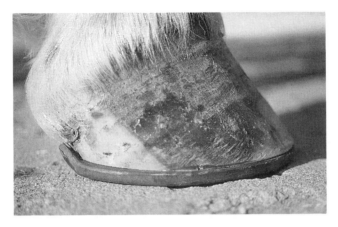

Properly fitted spooned heel shoes

CHAPTER 16

Teamwork

Your horse's performance should be the result of a team effort. You are the captain and must take responsibility for coordinating the efforts of the other players: the manager, the trainer, the instructor, the rider, the veterinarian and the farrier.

The Horse Your horse has no say in who is on his team, let alone where he lives, how he eats or what he does for a living. He is dependent on you to make wise decisions for him and to select the very best team members to assist him in his performance.

The Owner The owner is responsible for providing competent care and management of the horse, which includes feed, housing, exercise, veterinary and farrier care, grooming and proper training. When any of these duties are entrusted to another person, it is still the owner's responsibility to see that things are done correctly.

The Manager If you board your horse away from home or have hired someone to perform management chores at your barn, that person is essentially your horse's manager. He or she is responsible for seeing that your horse is safe, well fed and comfortable. The list of management tasks is quite long and encompasses everything from keeping the horse's blankets clean to being sure he has enough water to drink (see Recommended Reading in the Appendix). Specific to this book, the manager must be sure the horse's daily environment and management routines result in healthy hooves.

The Trainer The trainer is responsible not only for teaching the horse the specific performance requirements of his event, but also good ground manners as well. It is the trainer's responsibility to teach the horse the lessons outlined in Chapter 12 so the horse is relaxed and comfortable with shoeing procedures and is safe to work around. The trainer must work closely with the manager to thwart the formation of any bad habits or vices.

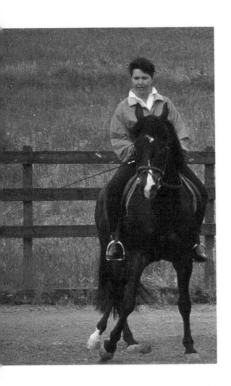

The trainer is not only responsible for teaching a horse the requirements of his sport but . . .

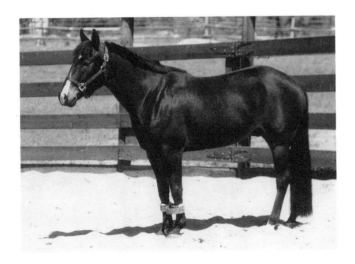

. . . also for teaching the horse manners and restraint (the same horse as in the previous photograph).

The Instructor The instructor's responsibility is to train the rider to be a good athlete when on horseback and not encumber the horse's movement. Part of the instructor's role is to preserve (and possibly enhance) the horse's level of training by increasing the rider's awareness of the various aspects of the horse's performance (see Recommended Reading in the Appendix).

The Rider The rider must dedicate herself to practicing effective, balanced riding. She must strive to be adept and coordinated through the various aspects of her horse's performance. When the horse exhibits a problem, the rider must first correct any deficiencies in riding. In this regard she works closely with her trainer, instructor and farrier in resolving any difficulties (see Recommended Reading in the Appendix).

The Veterinarian The veterinarian helps manage a horse's overall health as well as his limb and hoof soundness. Employ the services of a qualified equine veterinarian who keeps current on research, shoeing techniques and lameness diagnosis and treatment. Encourage your veterinarian to interact with your farrier. The combination of their knowledge and experience will benefit both you and your horse. Contact your veterinarian for advice and treatment related to lameness, wounds, foal hoof management and nutrition. Whenever a hoof injury involves sensitive tissue (hot nail, puncture, abscess, bleeding crack, coronary wound), it is important that your veterinarian be involved in the treatment. Although your farrier may perform the actual work (paring an abscess, relieving or resecting a crack, treating a hot nail), it should be done under a veterinarian's supervision.

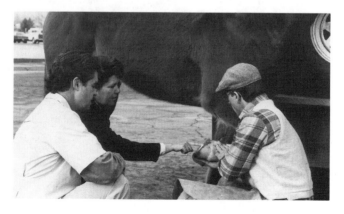

It is best if both your veterinarian and farrier are involved in a pre-purchase exam.

Your veterinarian and farrier should both be involved in pre-purchase evaluations and in helping you formulate a management program.

The Farrier The farrier's primary role is to trim and shoe the horse as naturally as possible, keeping principles of balance in mind. The farrier's goals should be (1) long-term soundness and (2) optimum performance. In addition, your farrier can assist your veterinarian, to the extent of his experience, in the treatment of various hoof and limb problems (Chapter 11). Ask your farrier to participate in pre-purchase examinations because his specialized hoof experience might allow him to spot hoof problems or tendencies missed by a veterinarian.

HOW TO FIND AND KEEP A GOOD FARRIER

Which farrier will best suit your needs depends on your level of riding, your event, your horse's specific shoeing requirements, which farriers are available and your budget. Because you want to give your horse the best care possible, secure the services of the most qualified farrier that you can afford.

What Makes a Good Farrier?

A good farrier is a true craftsman, one who has a genuine interest in the well-being of horses and pride in his work. He looks upon each hoof that he prepares and shoes as one that will bear his trademark and demonstrate the quality of his work. A keen farrier wants to keep informed about the latest research and developments in hoof care technology. A farrier that does not stay updated is outdated.

Because a farrier must usually be the secretary, accountant, and chief laborer in his small business, he must be a good manager of time. The successful farrier is dependable about keeping appointments. A farrier who is routinely late can cause inconvenience and frustration for horse owners, and such negligence can result in irregular care for the horses. A farrier must be careful to not pack his day so full that he gets in a hurry to keep on schedule, because then he will not do his best work. With one frantic day after another, there is no time to respond to emergencies or replace lost shoes.

A good farrier understands and is comfortable using standard methods of horse handling on a variety of horses. Although it is important to stay flexible regarding specific practices at various barns, it is a sign of a good farrier if he will not consent to work in unsafe conditions or on an untrained horse.

A good horseshoer should be able to accurately explain hoof care principles to horse owners. You should be able to ask your farrier what thrush is and how to deal with it and get a thorough, intelligent and accurate answer. His area of expertise is supposed to be the health and care of the hooves. If the answer to your question is "Thrush is that black gook and you don't want it," then you haven't really learned anything you didn't already know. Although your farrier doesn't have the time to teach you everything he has learned, he should be able to give you a good answer and then refer you to books or articles that deal with the topics that concern or interest you.

Just as there are all levels of horsemen, there are all levels of practicing horseshoers, from very basic, self-taught individuals to thoroughly educated, high-tech farriers. Horses with abnormal hooves or dramatic performance demands require the experience and skill of a top-notch farrier. When an inexperienced horseshoer is faced with quarter cracks, rununder heels, laminitis or navicular syndrome, he may not know what to do, and what he tries may make the situation worse. A good farrier is open minded and motivated, so that he seeks out and listens to advice when he is faced with a situation he or the other team members cannot resolve.

The greater the performance demands on a horse, the more precise his shoeing must be. The backyard pleasure horse with normal hooves may get along very well with shoes put on by a farrier who has only basic (but acceptable) skills. However, when that horse is sliding in the reining pen, turning the barrels, negotiating a jumper course or competing in an endurance ride, his shoeing requirements have become more specialized.

A horse may be able to accommodate to poor hoof care and improper shoeing for several months or even a few years. But be assured—the time that his feet are subjected to neglect and poor care will be subtracted from the end of his career . . . with interest.

As with anything else, you tend to get what you pay for in farrier service. Although the price of a standard shoeing (four keg shoes) can vary from well over $100 to less than $25, the national average is about $50. Prices vary regionally, with West Coast farrier fees being the highest, followed by the Southeast, the East Coast, the Midwest, the West, and the Southwest. Within a region, the variation in prices among farriers will be based on their level of experience, education, skill, demand, and location.

Finding a Good Farrier

If you need to find a farrier, use a combination of the following methods to identify the farrier most suitable to your needs.

Solicit recommendations. Ask five to ten people who they would recommend as a farrier. Try to get opinions from veterinarians, trainers, other horse owners and barn managers. Beginning with your own veterinarian, find out which farriers he has worked with, how capable the farrier was in solving problems, and if the farrier worked well with the owner in developing a good hoof management program. Ask your veterinarian not only to name the farriers he recommends but also those he does *not* recommend. Ask several other veterinarians in your area for their recommendations as well.

Ask some professional trainers, instructors, stable managers and breeders in your community which farriers they have had experiences with and which ones they currently employ. But don't rely on *one* person's opinion so strongly that you automatically hire or discredit a farrier. Just keep summarizing your findings, paying attention to details such as "He's really nice but he's never on time," or "My horses are always ready to step right into the show ring," or "He always gets in a fight with my horse." Ask how long it takes for various farriers to replace lost shoes; if a horse has ever been lame right after shoeing and what the farrier did about it; if the farrier works well with the farm veterinarian; if the farrier gets along well with horses.

Talk with horse owners who are like you. If you are a casual trail rider, it would be inappropriate to ask the rider of Grand Prix jumping horses for a farrier recommendation. Instead, find people who follow the same level of management that you do and who ride as frequently as you do in similar activities and ask them the same kinds of questions that you asked the professionals.

Read advertisements, but don't rely solely on them because many of the best farriers only use word-of-mouth advertising. Although some farriers you see advertised on bulletin boards or in papers might be very qualified, others could be very poorly qualified, no matter what their ads say, and they may create long-term problems for you and your horse.

Refer to farrier directories. Some countries require farriers to pass a government-regulated licensing program in order to practice. Currently in the United States, anyone can call himself a farrier. There is no mandatory testing or licensing.

However, there are many horseshoeing programs throughout the U.S. Some are part of the curriculum at colleges and universities, while others are held at independent horseshoeing schools. The programs range in length from one week to one year or more. Most programs issue a certificate or diploma after a student has completed the course. Some farriers, after attending one of these programs, will list themselves as "certified farrier" (referring to the certificate of completion) or "graduate farrier" (referring to having graduated from a program). Yet the qualifications of two farriers who call themselves "certified farriers" could be as different as night and day.

To help standardize the ratings of U.S. farriers (whether or not they've attended a farrier school), two national organizations operate voluntary testing and certification programs: The American Farriers Association (AFA) and The Brotherhood of Working Farriers Association (BWFA). Applicants to either association are required to pass written and/or oral exams and demonstrate shoeing skills.

Currently there are three examination levels offered by the AFA:

The *AFA Intern Classification* indicates one who has graduated from formal horseshoeing training, has competed an apprenticeship or has otherwise progressed in elementary skills and knowledge of horseshoeing.

The *AFA Certified Farrier* candidate must have a minimum of one year of practical experience and must meet the basic standard of horseshoeing knowledge and skill to be designated a qualified farrier.

The *AFA Certified Journeyman Farrier* candidate must have a minimum of two years experience, must have passed the Certified Farrier examinations and must demonstrate a superior level of knowledge and skill related to horseshoeing.

The Brotherhood of Working Farriers Association (BWFA) offers five levels:

The *BWFA Apprentice I* candidate has less than six months of practical shoeing experience or has attended a two-week horseshoeing course.

The *BWFA Apprentice II* candidate has less than six months of practical shoeing experience or has attended a six- or eight-week horseshoeing course.

The *BWFA Journeyman I* candidate has more than six months practical shoeing experience but has little experience in hot shoeing.

The *BWFA Journeyman II* candidate has more than three years practical shoeing and forge experience.

The *BWFA Master Farrier* candidate must have been a Journeyman II farrier for at least four years, must have seven years practical shoeing and forge experience, and be a full-time farrier or must be a full-time farrier with fifteen years of shoeing and forge experience but with no previous certification.

Today the AFA Certified Journeyman Farrier designation is the most difficult U.S. certification to obtain because of the complexity of the written exam and the extensive shoe-making requirements in the practical exam.

Both associations maintain a directory of farriers' names, addresses, phone numbers, and level of certification. By contacting the AFA or BWFA (see Resource Guide in the Appendix) you can obtain the names of certified farriers in your area. Since membership and testing is voluntary, if you rely solely on the AFA or BWFA farrier list, you may miss finding a very talented and capable farrier who lives just down the road from you but isn't a member of either association.

Keeping the Good Farrier

Since scheduling is the most common problem in getting continuous farrier service, find out your farrier's preference for handling appointments. Does he schedule a definite appointment seven weeks in advance? If so, do you have to confirm the appointment the day before or do you both just show up? Does the farrier require the owner or someone to be present when he is working? What happens if one of you misses the appointment?

Some farriers prefer clients to call close to the time of shoeing to set up a specific appointment. If so, when should you call? Three weeks ahead or one day ahead?

When you are making an appointment, mention any special problems or needs that your horses may have so your shoer can have necessary supplies on hand when he visits. Although some farrier's trucks are veritable stores filled with an assortment of shoes, pads, nails, and accessories, other farriers like to travel light. If your horse has unusually large or small feet, needs studs, polo shoes, sliders, snow pads or requires quarter crack repair, let your farrier know. If you need to change your appointment, have the courtesy to call your farrier so he can adjust the rest of that day's schedule accordingly.

Discuss payment arrangements with your farrier. Some farriers use a monthly billing system, especially with larger barns or with clients who have a large number of horses. Others require payment at time of services, so if you will not be there in person, arrange to leave a check for the farrier. That way you will be ensured of continued farrier service.

All horses that are scheduled for work should be readily available when your farrier arrives. The horses can be tied or crosstied in the barn or in stalls or small pens conviently located to the working area.

The Work Area

To enable your farrier to do his very best work, provide him with a proper shoeing area and well-mannered horses (Chapter 12). Your farrier may have personal opinions about the type of floor he prefers or whether he likes to work in a small enclosure or a large open area. However, there are certain criteria that must be met for any shoeing to proceed safely and efficiently.

The shoeing area should be well lighted, uncluttered and level. The flooring can be concrete, rubber, wood or asphalt; tile, very smooth concrete and some rubber mats can be slippery when wet. Your farrier should not be expected to shoe in a driveway, in the snow, out in the middle of a pasture, in a muddy or rocky paddock or in a dusty barn aisle. Gravel can damage a freshly trimmed hoof in a matter of seconds while the farrier is preparing the shoe. Shoeing in

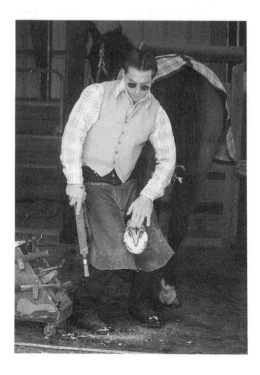

A good shoeing area

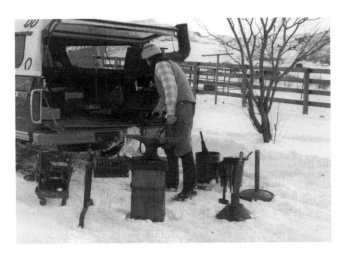

Undesirable shoeing area

a barn aisle full of potholes makes it very difficult for the farrier to accurately assess limb balance and often makes it difficult for the horses to stand squarely.

In temperate climates, there should be a well-lighted indoor shoeing area that is out of the snow and wind. During the summer and in the southern states, some farriers prefer to work in a shaded outdoor area where the breeze can keep the farrier and the horse cool. Since most farriers use electric tools for shoe preparation, the shoeing area should have access to 110-volt electrical outlets.

Some farriers prefer to have horses held by an experienced horseman when they shoe. It is best if the handler stands on the opposite side of the farrier. This keeps the horse from moving away from the farrier. Other farriers would rather work on the horse tied at a hitching post or in crossties. The tie area should be strong and safe. When tied at a hitching post, the horse should be tied at or above the level of the withers with approximately 2 to 3 feet of rope between the halter and the post. A shorter rope prevents the horse from attaining a comfortable head position and makes it difficult for the horse to move freely when asked by the farrier. A longer rope often allows the horse to lower his head too much and move his body around. The height of crossties will vary according to the width of the alley spanned. Very wide alleys require long crossties that must be mounted high; crossties in narrow alleys are shorter and can be mounted so that the ties aim almost horizontally at the cheekpieces of the horse's halter.

If your horses have come out of muddy lots, be sure to clean them, especially their shoulders, hindquarters and legs, which come into contact with the farrier. Also, scrape and then wipe the mud off the hooves rather than hosing them off. Clean, dry hooves are much safer and more pleasant for the farrier to work on than slippery, wet hooves. Be sure your horses are well mannered for shoeing (Chapter 12).

One of the best ways to keep a good farrier is to be genuinely interested in the health of your horse's hooves. Be a conscientious manager and rider and learn all you can about hoof care and shoeing. The more knowledgeable you are, the better able you will be to converse with your farrier. Stay informed by reading specialized articles related to shoeing.

The care of your horse's hooves is a team effort. Take the time to find a really interested, skilled farrier, then treat him like the professional he is and you will likely be able to retain his good services.

Here's to Maximum Hoof Power.

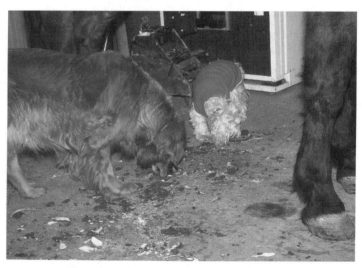

Dogs should not be allowed in the work area.

- *Do* offer to hold your horses rather than tie them if it is their first time for trimming or shoeing, but
  Don't feel offended if your offer is rejected. Your farrier may prefer to work alone with the horse tied.
- *Do* have plenty of fly repellent on hand, but
  Don't wait until your farrier's visit to acquaint your horse with a spray bottle, and
  Don't spray the horse while your farrier is working under him.
- *Do* introduce your dogs to your farrier, but
  Don't let your dogs roam loose where the farrier is working.
- *Do* tell your horseshoer the name, age and use of each horse, but
  Don't tell about each ribbon he's won, the time he jumped the fence, the first time you showed him a pig. . . . You shouldn't expect your farrier to really listen to you or to carry on a conversation because he is there for one reason—to provide a professional service that allows you to participate in your favorite horse activities. The less attention he has to give you, the more he can give to the work you are paying for.
- *Do* pay attention to your horse's behavior, but
  Don't take your nervous horse for a hike down the gravel driveway on freshly trimmed feet while the farrier is shaping a shoe.
- *Do* discuss stable management and hoof care with your farrier. Ask him about the symptoms of problems he may see in your horse's feet and listen to his recommendations for remedying them, but
  Don't expect miracles from your farrier. If you bought a horse that had been neglected for two years, or if you have a horse with crooked legs, or if you board at a stable with muddy pens, don't think that your farrier has a magic rasp that can cure cracks, founder, conformation flaws or thrush. You must work together toward gradual, permanent results.
- *Do* have your payment in full ready before he leaves;
  Don't make him ask.
- *Do* offer him a place to wash up and a glass of water, and
  Don't forget to write down the date for your next appointment.

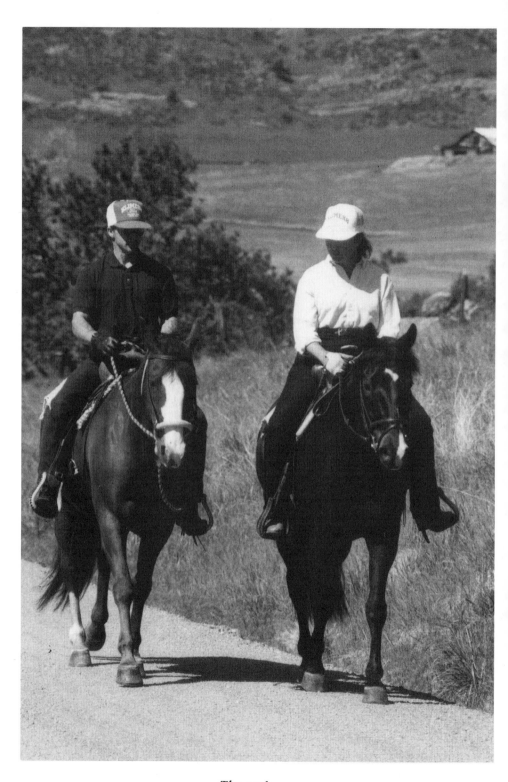

The authors

Appendix

RECOMMENDED BOOKS

Butler, Doug, PhD., *The Principles of Horseshoeing II*, LaPorte, CO:
    Doug Butler Publisher, 1985.
Camarillo, Sharon, *Barrel Racing*, Colorado Springs, CO:
    Western Horseman Books, 1985.
Carpenter, Doug, *Western Pleasure*, Austin: Equimedia, 1996.
deKunffy, Charles, *The Athletic Development of the Dressage Horse*, Foster City, CA:
    IDG Books Worldwide, 1992.
Dunning, Al, *Reining*, Revised, Colorado Springs, CO: Western Horseman
    Books, 1996.
Harrell, Leon, *Cutting*, Colorado Springs, CO: Western Horseman Books, 1990.
Harris, Susan E., *Horse Gaits, Balance and Movement*, Foster City, CA: IDG Books
    Worldwide, 1993.
Heymering, Henry, *On the Horse's Foot, Shoes and Shoeing: the Bibliographic
    Record*, Cascade, MO: St. Eloy Publishing, 1990.
Hill, Cherry, *Becoming An Effective Rider*, Pownal, VT: Storey Books, 1991.
    The Formative Years, Ossining, NY: Breakthrough, 1988
    From the Center of the Ring, An Inside View of Horse Competitions,
    Pownal, VT: Storey Books, 1988.
    Horse Health Care, Pownal, VT: Storey Books, 1997.
    Horse Handling and Grooming, Pownal, VT: Storey Books, 1997.
    Horse for Sale, Foster City, CA: IDG Books Worldwide, 1995.
    Horsekeeping on a Small Acreage, Pownal, VT: Storey Books, 1990.
    Making Not Breaking, Ossining NY: Breakthrough, 1992.
    Stablekeeping, Pownal, VT: Storey Books, 2000.
    Trailering Your Horse, Pownal, VT: Storey Books, 2000.
Jackson, Jaime, *Horse Owners Guide to Natural Hoof Care*, Harrison, AR: Star
    Ridge Publishing, 1999.

Krolick, David, *Shoeing Right*, Ossining, NY: Breakthrough, 1992.

Lewis, Lon D., *Feeding and Care of the Horse*, 2nd edition, Fairfield, NJ: Login Brothers Book Co., 1995.

Loomis, Bob, *Reining*, Austin: Equimedia, 1990.

Stashak, Ted, DVM and Hill, Cherry, *Practical Guide to Lameness in Horses*, Philadelphia: Lippincott, Williams & Wilkins, 1995.

Wright, Ed, *Barrel Racing*, Austin: Equimedia, 1999.

FARRIER PUBLICATIONS

American Farriers Journal, PO Box 624, Brookfield, WI 53008-0624, info@lesspub.com, www.lesspub.com/afj (*official journal of the American Farriers Association*).

Anvil, PO Box 1810, Georgetown, CA 95634-1810, anvil@anvilmag.com, www.anvilmag.com (*practical articles on horseshoeing and blacksmithing*).

European Farriers Journal, 16, rue d'Opprebais, B 1360 Malèves-Sainte-Marie, Belgium, Tel. int. + 32 (0) 10 88 88 98, Info@farriersjournal.com, http://www.farriersjournal.com (*bimonthly international magazine*)

Hoofcare & Lameness: Journal of Equine Foot Science, PO Box 6600, Gloucester, MA 01930, franjurga@aol.com, www.hoofcare.com (*practical articles and research on farrier science*).

FARRIER ORGANIZATIONS

American Farriers Association, 4059 Iron Works Pkwy, Suite 2, Lexington, KY 40511; (606) 233-7411, farriers@aol.com, www.amfarriers.com

Brotherhood of Working Farriers Association, 14013 East Highway 136, LaFayette, GA 30728; (706) 397-8047, farrierhdq@aol.com, www.bwfa.net

Guild of Professional Farriers, PO Box 684, Locust, NC 28097, (301) 898-6990, theguild@horseshoes.com, www.horseshoes.com/theguild/

RESOURCE GUIDE

Centaur Forge Ltd., P.O. Box 340, Burlington, WI 53105, (414) 763-9175, centforge1@aol.com, www.centaurforge.com (*farrier books, videos, tools, and supplies, shoe size comparison chart*).

Equilox International, PO Box 428A, Pine Island, MN 55963, (800) 551-4394, equilox123@aol.com, www.equilox.com (*Equilox, prosthetic hoof repair material*).

Farrier and Hoofcare Resource Center, 1265 Ash Lane, Lebanon, PA 17042, (717) 279-6666, horseshoes@horshoes.com, www.horseshoes.com (*online hoof care articles, discussion groups, consultation, products, schools, organizations)*

Glu-Strider, PO Box 7315, Bloomfield, CT 06002, (203) 726-1927, info@mustadinc.com, www.mustadinc,com (*glue on-shoes*).

Hawthorne Products Inc., Box 66, RD 2, Dunkirk, IN 47336, (800) 548-5658, drhobso@ibm.net, www.hawthorne-products.com (*hoof packing*).

High Performance Horse Products, Farnam Companies Inc., PO Box 34820, Phoenix, AZ 85067-4820, (800) 327-9792, info@mail.farnam.com, http://www.farnam.com/division_horse/proequine.html (*Pro Equine protective horse boots*).

Klimesh, Richard, Video: *Welding Clips with a Wire-Feed Welder*, P.O. Box 140, Livermore, CO, 80536, (970) 221-2948, rklimesh@horsekeeping.com (*applying clips for preventive and therapeutic use; includes the Klimesh Contiguous Clip Shoe, and heel shields*).

Level-It, 10235 W. Sample Road, Suite 207, Coral Springs, FL 33065, (800) 408-2900, llevel-it@aol.com, http://www.horseshoes.com/supplies (*material for hoof leveling, balancing and repair*)

Life Data Labs, Inc., P.O. Box 490, Cherokee, AL 35616 (800) 624-1873, msgravlee@lifedatalabs.com, http://www.lifedatalabs.com (*Farrier's Formula hoof supplement*).

Index

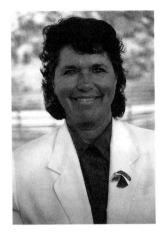

Cherry Hill is the author of over 1,000 articles and twenty-three books on horse training and care. In 1992, Cherry was awarded first place by the American Horse Publications for editorial excellence in Service to the Reader for her work in the *American Farrier's Journal.* In 1994 she received the American Farriers Association's Journalism Award for meritorious service in collecting, editing, and presenting information of interest to farriers. Cherry taught university courses in riding, training, and management in the US and Canada for ten years and has been a horse show judge for over twenty years.

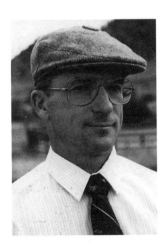

Richard Klimesh is a Journeyman Farrier with the American Farriers Association, a Registered Farrier with the Guild of Professional Farriers and a Master Farrier with the Brotherhood of Working Farriers and was a practicing farrier for seventeen years. He provided therapeutic shoeing for Colorado State University Veterinary Teaching Hospital and also had a clientele of performance horses: reiners, hunters, jumpers, dressage, cutters, ropers, barrel racers, police and endurance. With his wife Cherry Hill, he is currently working on books and articles and is developing a series of videotapes on horse care and training.